TAKING CARE OF OUR OWN

A volume in the series
THE CULTURE AND POLITICS OF HEALTH CARE WORK
Edited by Suzanne Gordon and Sioban Nelson

For a list of books in the series, visit our website at cornellpress.cornell.edu.

Taking Care of Our Own

When Family Caregivers Do Medical Work

Sherry N. Mong

ILR Press

an imprint of

Cornell University Press

Ithaca and London

First published 2020 by Cornell University Press

Library of Congress Cataloging-in-Publication Data

Names: Mong, Sherry N., 1961– author.
Title: Taking care of our own : when family caregivers do medical work / Sherry N. Mong.
Description: Ithaca [New York] : Cornell University Press, 2020. | Series: The culture and politics of health care work | Includes bibliographical references and index.
Identifiers: LCCN 2019056309 (print) | LCCN 2019056310 (ebook) | ISBN 9781501751448 (hardcover) | ISBN 9781501751455 (paperback) | ISBN 9781501751479 (pdf) | ISBN 9781501751462 (epub)
Subjects: LCSH: Caregivers—Social conditions. | Home care services—Social aspects. | Unpaid labor—Social aspects.
Classification: LCC RA645.3. M655 2020 (print) | LCC RA645.3 (ebook) | DDC 362.14—dc23
LC record available at https://lccn.loc.gov/2019056309
LC ebook record available at https://lccn.loc.gov/2019056310

To Alan, Andi, and Colin
And caregivers, care recipients, and home health nurses everywhere

CONTENTS

Acknowledgments

It's hard to express what the journey of writing this book has meant in my life and in the lives of my family. What started as a personal family experience has been transformed by understanding more about the work of scholars who have paved paths before me, and the experiences of others. I am forever grateful for all those who took the time to speak with me about their perspectives and experiences with skilled home health labor. I have done my best to honor these insights and weave them into a fuller understanding of the labor processes that occur.

I thank Steven Lopez for his kindness, insight, and encouragement. As my mentor at Ohio State University (OSU), Steve never wavered in his view that my writings should be turned into a book, and he reviewed and gave feedback on all the revisions. Steve has an uncanny ability to look at all angles of a research question and cut through to the heart of it. He provided emotional support and guidance, listened to and honed my ideas, and told me I was doing a "great job" at just the moments I needed to hear it. His humor, candor, and genuine spirit were resources for me and provided sparks of optimism during the long book process. He never gave up on me.

I also thank Vincent Roscigno and Liana Sayer, both of whom reviewed drafts of the manuscript. Vinnie provided countless days of counsel and guidance at OSU. I found him to be one of the most understanding people I have ever worked with, and I am grateful for his thoughtful style, caring nature, and mentorship. Liana was always willing to stop and talk. She often asked how I was doing, and listened as I recounted the latest updates. Liana provided feedback and encouragement, and I sincerely appreciate her guidance. There are many other people in the OSU Sociology Department that deserve my thanks and recognition. The members of Steven Lopez's qualitative writing class reviewed early versions of the manuscript. Other colleagues offered support and kindness, including Susan Ortiz, Eileen E. Avery, Lisette Garcia, and office mates Jill Harrison and Justin Schupp.

At Capital University, I have also enjoyed meaningful relationships with colleagues who have offered encouragement, including Tracy Roberts, Basil Kardaras, Laura Kane, Andrea Karkowski, Nate Jackson, Stephanie Wilson, Kathryn Bell, Deanna Wagner, Suzanne Marilley, and Janette McDonald. I am fortunate to be part of a learning community that values collegiality and thinks critically about social justice issues. My students also continue to inspire me with their engagement, passion, and application of knowledge, and I look forward to seeing the good they will do.

This book would never have become a reality if it were not for Suzanne Gordon at ILR Press/Cornell. I appreciate her immeasurable guidance and astute feedback. Suzanne challenged me at every step to make the book more relatable and readable. She encouraged me to use my voice in order to craft a clearer path through the literature and the data. Sioban Nelson was also an integral part of the process and gave invaluable input in her review of the manuscript. She stated her views candidly and kindly. Clare Stacey's comments challenged me to develop the emotional labor sections, and to more fully integrate and frame the data. I am grateful for these scholars. I also appreciate editorial guidance from Mary Kate Murphy and Fran Benson, and Eric Levy's fine attention to detail elevated the manuscript considerably.

I also greatly appreciate partial funding received for this project, including a Dissertation Grant from the OSU Department of Sociology; the

Alumni Grant for Graduate Research and Scholarship Dissertation Grant from the OSU Graduate School; and the Coca-Cola Critical Difference for Women Graduate Studies Grant for Research on Women, Gender, or Gender Equity from the OSU Department of Women's Studies.

As evidenced by my experiences, no scholar makes contributions alone. My personal friends and family were also incredibly supportive throughout the process. Barb Breth and Beth Wepprich listened to me on many occasions, and Monesa and Chris Skocik's hospitality during times when I had worked long hours was an incredible gift. My mother, Iva Newcomb, as always, was a source of emotional support and quiet strength. My sister, Terry Newcomb, provided immeasurable support—even document formatting and reference checking—during the book publication process. My mother- and father-in-law, Eloise and Neil Mong, provided emotional support and hands-on help with childcare and errands during my years of research. My children, Andi and Colin, were also extremely supportive of the process and always understood when I needed to work. Andi even used her incredible organizational skills to catalog and file journal articles for me. Most importantly, I thank my best friend, and life partner, Alan Mong. Without him, I could not have found my passion and might not have known how to look for it. In multiple ways—through conversations, encouragement, even hands-on help, including computer assistance—he has been a constant source of strength and support throughout these years. Thank you, Alan.

Taking Care of Our Own

INTRODUCTION

On the day I brought my three-and-a-half-year-old son home from his first hospital stay, I sat in the big oak rocker in our family room, taking a single moment to reflect on the sights and sounds around me. I looked out the window. It was nice outside. Sun drenched the dark green meadows that surrounded the house and I imagined onlookers on their way home or to work, taking notice of the peaceful scenery. As I rocked back and forth, I considered the commotion in the room around me. In contrast to the flowing meadows, inside there was an entirely different landscape—a landscape with rocky terrain and blurred boundaries. A landscape riddled by uncertainty.

My son, who has cystic fibrosis, had just finished his first hospital admission for a lung infection. The day before, the hospital resident had explained to me that "most parents" of children with cystic fibrosis administer IV antibiotics at home. That way, their child is released from the hospital sooner and is not exposed to the bacteria that often plague hospital wards. It seemed logical, and I had desperately wanted to do the right thing for my son. I was not working outside the home at the time, and my husband, a physician, had long hours at work. We had agreed that I would stay home while the kids were young, and return to pursue a master's degree once they reached school age. In that situation I seemed the "natural" person to do the care. But I now realized that I had no real concept of what this new kind of care would mean for me.

I could barely register the actions of the home health nurses and family members around me. More vividly I remember the mess of tubing, wires, IV poles, and bags that were draped in half-opened boxes about the family room. I walked over to the couch to join the nurse. She began talking directly to me. She was kind but stern. She had long, straight hair, and I remember thinking her earthy look somehow clashed with the severity of the situation. She told me it was important to draw up the saline now so that it could be refrigerated for future use. That way, she said, I wouldn't have to be bothered with it every time I administered the IV antibiotics.

As I was trying to focus my thoughts, she showed me how to uncap the syringe, draw air into it, plunge it into the saline bottle, push the syringe to release the air into the bottle, and pull back. If any air bubbles formed in the syringe, as they most certainly would, I was to flick the syringe with my thumb and middle finger to break them up. Next she showed me how to manipulate the syringe so I could shoot out the excess air before recapping it. It was extremely important, she said, not to touch the surface of the bottle or the tip of the needle with my fingers. Cautiously I performed the duties, more than once spewing saline into the air as I struggled to shoot the excess air out of the syringe. The first time made me gasp, but she seemed unconcerned, so I learned to watch the unpredictable fountains as they shot straight up then cascaded down and out before landing on the carpet and furniture. She then instructed me to perform the same procedures with the heparin. I complied, while she observed me.

She asked if I had any gallon-sized plastic bags. I said I did. Following her advice, I labeled the bags with a big *S* or *H* using a black permanent marker. We then placed the freshly prepared saline and heparin syringes into the respective bags. She said this would help ensure that I didn't get the doses mixed up when I needed them in the middle of the night. We went to the refrigerator. On the shelf directly under our usual stock of milk and orange juice, we placed the saline and heparin bags beside several other prepackaged bags of antibiotics. Until that moment, I hadn't realized that "hospital things" had any place alongside my ketchup and mayonnaise. It was an odd combination; the placement seemed unnatural and unsettling.

I slowly made my way back to the rocker—a place of seeming refuge in my quiet, private chaos. I remember sitting dumbly, still in a head fog, as the nurse spelled out the formula to administer the antibiotics. "S . . . A . . . S . . . H," she told me. "Saline, antibiotic, saline, heparin." I repeated the command, but in the rush around me, I had hundreds of unformed thoughts flying like fireflies in the meadow outside. I felt a deep sense of confusion. I was afraid, and worried in a way I could not explain.

I had been an accountant by trade. On that first day of at-home nurse's training, two themes permeated my otherwise scattered thinking. First, I had never been to nursing school. I had no medical training and no inclination whatsoever toward the medical profession. Surely I wasn't the best person to administer IVs to my son. What if I made a mistake? What if I hurt him? What if something went horribly wrong? How would I be able to handle a situation like that? Second, I believed the training I did have to be virtually useless. Though I was well educated, my prior work and personal experience were inadequate in preparing me for the tasks that day or the ones that would certainly lie ahead. Accounting was as polar an opposite as one could imagine from administering IV antibiotics. Mothering, while giving me skills to work through a myriad of child-rearing issues, from fixing "boo-boos" to instilling personal values, gave me no help at all on how to perform this type of medical procedure. Surely this process—whatever it was—was way beyond mothering.

And so I felt I lacked a knowledge base from which to formulate the feelings I had. My own thoughts were not even sufficiently developed enough for me to express myself. Although I didn't know it at the time, I was standing in a situation akin to what Dorothy Smith (1987, 49) has described as a "line of fault": a "rupture" between my experiences and "the social forms of consciousness—the culture or ideology of . . . society."[1] Foremost, I wanted to be a good mother. But the skills I needed to learn required much more timing, precision, and training than the typical housework or care work I had ever done or known about. In housework, as in child rearing, I could decide what was right, and go at my own pace. Now I was being judged on something totally different. I was being asked to perform a medical procedure, which was more in the scope of registered nursing than mothering. And the stakes were very high. I knew that I had to do everything right, or it could have huge implications for the health of my son. I also had the responsibility of conveying to him that this was the right thing to do. I needed to let him know that this would be part of his life, and was in fact meant to help him. I did not want him to be afraid.

But nagging questions continued to haunt me. Was it appropriate that I should be doing these types of procedures for my own son? Was I competent to do them? What was my role here? Would the stress of giving my son IVs interfere with my ability to care for him by just being his mom? Would I be able to give him the emotional support he needed while dealing with my own feelings of anxiety? Further, he had left the hospital with a peripheral IV in his arm. Should it come loose, the home health nurse would have to stick him again with a large needle. Shouldn't home be a place of comfort and hospitals the place for needles and blood draws? I longed to run to the meadows outside and escape the shaky terrain within. Surely someone else could do a better job of this than I could.

But on that day, as on all the rest, my desire to be a "good mother" won out over the fear that threatened to paralyze me. I didn't bolt, but stayed and learned the procedures. And through the years, with bouts of required antibiotics, sometimes running two to three IV lines up to four times a day, for periods lasting up to two weeks, on top of regular cystic fibrosis treatments, such as breathing treatments and chest physical therapy, I did the job. These were, indeed, intense periods of exhaustion and little sleep. During most of it, especially the first several runs, I was racked with anxiety. I checked and rechecked my work. I pored over my notes. I constantly reorganized medicines to get a better handle on things, and through it all, I was still subtly terrified. Were it not for my family and my husband, who not only was a wonderful resource but also shared the actual work with me when he was not at his job, I'm sure things would have been much more difficult. While I know that I am very privileged in this regard,[2] it is also true that many of my experiences with home health care were often alone, when my husband was unavailable or called away.

During those times, trying to run IV lines in my son's bedroom at night, awkwardly uncapping, injecting, remembering S . . . A . . . S . . . H, while taking care not to wake him, I often wondered about the experiences of others who are in similar situations. Indeed, my curiosity led to a fundamental concern to understand more about what other caregivers go through when they learn skilled medical labor. What kind of procedures do they have to learn? What is the process like for them? Do they, too, have a rough time processing their new duties? Are their problems like mine, or different? My desire to find answers to these types of questions—questions embedded in the social processes of what philosophers such as Kittay (1999, 29) call the "human condition"—was a fundamental reason for my decision to go to graduate school and study sociology. My training as a sociologist led me to work by C. Wright Mills (1959), and in Mills's terms, I wanted to use my "sociological imagination" to understand how my personal troubles were linked to troubles in the lives of others. According to Mills, if I could find linkages, I would have a greater understanding of the public issues related to skilled home health care—issues that affect society at large.

And so I wanted to know how family caregivers deal—both emotionally and physically—with the skilled nursing they perform. I wanted to hear their stories and understand more about what they go through. I wanted to know whether they, at least initially, were as bewildered as I had been. I also wanted to talk to the nurses who teach the labor. I wanted to find out how they show others how to perform these procedures, and I wanted to see the home health process through their eyes. As a result, between January 2009 and February 2010, I conducted sixty-two in-depth semi-structured interviews in two midwestern states. (See the appendix for a complete discussion of methods used.) I was able to learn from people who are directly involved in the process, and I believe that, taken together, these stories provide rich insight into how home health labor is enacted in the lives of women and men. Importantly, while theirs are not my stories, my experiences certainly are relevant and no doubt contribute to the work I do, as I attempt to look beyond the green meadows that surround our visions of "home life" and capture instead glimpses of the terrain inside.

The Debate over Home Health Care

At first glance, at-home skilled nursing seems a natural result of medical advancement in a technological age. People are now able to access medical information about their illnesses on the internet. They can live at home on portable oxygen. They can inject themselves with IV medications—something that was impossible fifty years ago. Moreover, home health advocates—including home health agency managers, lobbyists, and many medical professionals—contend that patients are happiest and heal best in their homes, away from hospital distractions, multiple caregivers, and other patients, all of which can increase infection rates and reduce quality of care. Proponents also point to the dignity and independence that care recipients enjoy at home, as well as the immense cost savings of using home health care over institutionalization (NAHC 2019).

Those critical of the push toward at-home skilled caregiving have focused on these cost-saving policies, seeing them as an attempt to unload labor onto unpaid family members who have little recourse (Glazer 1993). Opponents contend that home health care is often touted as "cheaper," with no real consideration of caregiver costs. Cost-saving strategies have indeed been at the forefront of changes in Medicare and other payer sources, and this has meant that nursing agencies, which used to be able to do more of the skilled work, have been pressed to find effective ways of transferring medical tasks to families (see chapter 3). In a column on our self-service society, Ellen Goodman (2008) muses that we are now "expected to interact with 'labor-saving technology' without realizing that it's labor-transferring technology. . . . In an era when every operation short of brain surgery is done on an outpatient basis, nursing care has . . . been outsourced to family members whose entire medical training consists of TiVo-ing 'Grey's Anatomy.' "

So how are we to conceptualize skilled at-home nursing care and its effect on families in contemporary society? To analyze the "home care is best" versus "caregivers primarily are forced laborers" viewpoints, we must first realize how they differ in their approach to skilled caregiving. The "home care is best" view casts the home as a place of rest and healing, and emphasizes the patient's comfort and the caregiver's love and concern.[3] This view, however, downplays the costs associated with caregiving. This is a large understatement. Scholars estimate that family caregivers provide hundreds of billions of dollars a year in unpaid labor,[4] and a survey by the National Alliance for Caregiving (NAC and Evercare 2007) estimates that caregivers spend an average of $5,500 per year—a figure that does not include their lost wages. My interviews with caregivers who have performed skilled care also reveal that they face many unmet needs. Sometimes nurses are able to stay only a short amount of time, and home life is often busy and filled with other obligations. There are issues with balancing work and family care, and many caregivers experienced sleeplessness and anxiety. Though most caregivers developed a "you do what you have to do" attitude and were able to figure out a way to perform the tasks, it was not a simple process.

The second viewpoint, which focuses on caregivers primarily as forced laborers, recognizes caregivers' labor, and the enormous contributions they make, but downplays the gratification that many have found in helping their loved ones, as well as the nuances of the caregiver–care recipient relationship. Under a strict interpretation of this viewpoint, caregivers seem more like victims than anything else. Many of the caregivers I spoke with were ready to leave the hospitals or rehab facilities with their loved ones, and preferred to be in familiar and comfortable surroundings. Overall, many also expressed that they wanted to take care of their loved ones, and said they felt deep satisfaction in their caregiving labor.

Indeed, these important components of caregiving—that it involves both labor and love as well as satisfaction and costs—have been recognized and addressed by care work scholars (Abel and Nelson 1990; Abel 1991; Graham 1983). Abel and Nelson (1990, 6–7) state that socialist feminist views that focus on the material and ideological mechanisms that oblige women to provide care, as well as feminist views that emphasize the humanizing aspects and personal fulfillment of caregiving, are both inadequate. The first, they say, leave out human connectedness, while the second run the danger of contributing to women's subordination (1990, 7). While Glazer's (1993) work—which viewed the "work transfer" on a Marxist scale and called attention to the structural processes that place nursing care on caregivers—was incredibly important, it did not consider important microprocesses such as caregivers' own interpretations of their labor, the identities of care workers, and the interactions and relationships between caregivers, care recipients, and nurses.

These insights tell us that the panacea-like home care rhetoric and the forced labor scenario are both oversimplifications. "Home care for all" downplays caregiver labor and does not consider unmet caregiver needs or the particular nuisances of the home health situation. Seeing caregivers mainly as forced laborers, however, denies the agency of those who genuinely want to help their loved ones when they need them most. An honest assessment of skilled home care should recognize interactional components as well as structural constraints, while remembering that caregiving involves both labor and love (Abel and Nelson 1990; Graham 1983).

Indeed, scholars are increasingly recognizing the multifaceted nature of caregiving, and the fact that care work itself entails intrinsic rewards as well as costs and obligations (see, for example, Folbre and Wright 2012). An expansive body of work on caregiving documents the associated stresses and burdens (see Bianchi, Folbre, and Wolf 2012), and shows that caregivers have less time for rest and exercise (Burton et al. 1997), give up leisure time, and report increased financial costs, including out-of-pocket expenses (Leonard, Brust, and Sapienza 1992; NAC and Evercare 2007). A host of studies also show that caregiving is associated with depressive symptoms and psychological distress (Schulz et al. 1995; Cannuscio et al. 2004; Hirst 2005), worse physical health (Pinquart and Sörensen 2007), and perceived ill health (NAC and AARP 2009).[5]

Despite these costs, however, studies have also shown that caregiving can have positive benefits, such as increased closeness to loved ones, a sense of satisfaction regarding the importance of the care, and improved mental health (Elmore 2014, 18–19).[6] Green (2007) found that caregivers of children with disabilities experienced a sense of strength, closer family relationships, and an ability to look beyond appearances. In a national study, Donelan and colleagues (2002) found that 71 percent of informal caregivers said their relationship with their care recipient had improved, and 89 percent said their care recipient had expressed appreciation for what they had done. Such studies paint a picture of caregiving as multifaceted and deeply rooted in social relationships (see Abel 1991).

It is clear that we need further assessment of the daily work processes enacted in homes and a better understanding of how caregivers experience these processes—both emotionally and physically. Such an assessment is critical in the midst of increasing technology and demographic changes that significantly impact home health care, including an increase in the elderly population, smaller families that are more geographically dispersed, a large growth in the adult population living alone, and the fact that only around 3.5 percent of adults over age sixty-five are in institutional care (Glenn 2010; Moeller 2013; USDHHS 2013).[7]

Drawing on feminist, medical sociology, and care work literature (see, for example, Daniels 1987; Corbin and Strauss 1988; Abel and Nelson 1990; James 1992; Glazer 1993; Bolton 2000; Cancian and Oliker 2000;

Folbre and Wright 2012; Duffy, Albelda, and Hammonds 2013; Erickson and Stacey 2013), a central tenet of this book is that the unpaid, skilled caregiving activities that are integral to the work in home health care need to be considered as "labor processes"—processes that include both emotional and physical/instrumental labor. Early studies of labor processes were performed in manufacturing settings, and offered detailed descriptions of methods that paid workers used to learn the work, workers' strategies and feelings about their labor, and their identity construction and consent to the labor process (Roy 1952; Braverman 1974; Burawoy 1979). In her 1993 work, Glazer refers to the "labor process" in describing the "work transfer," which takes place when women's unpaid labor becomes "decommodified" and structural forces create a labor force of paid and unpaid workers (215). Citing Braverman's (1974) use of the term "labor process,"[8] Folbre and Wright contend that studying the "labor process" in care work "calls attention to the lived experience of work and highlights the qualitative features of interactions among care managers, care providers, and care recipients" (2012, 5).

Using a labor process lens allows us to see caregivers' interactions and what they go through in their performance of everyday labor. How do they learn specific skills? What types of training do they receive? How do they make sense of their labor? How are emotions and relationships important? We are also able to understand how nurses teach this labor. How do they teach such complex skills to caregivers, and how do they feel about transferring their technical skills? Exploring and answering these and many more questions helps us understand how narrow both policy and personal choices are, and how we can analyze this new form of work in a way that recognizes both labor and love.[9]

Unpaid Care Work as Work

Interestingly, workplace scholars have generally confined their analyses of medical labor to paid wage labor.[10] Considering the abundance of labor studies that critique capitalism for its exploitative effects, the lack of attention given to unpaid labor is ironic.[11] By recognizing only those who are compensated, scholars allow capitalism to define work processes and to determine who it is that we consider as workers. Feminist scholars have convincingly shown that capitalism and labor markets themselves depend on unpaid labor (Glazer 1984, 1990; Daniels 1987; James 1989). Glenn (2010) makes the case that coercion by the state and capitalism place undue burdens on family caregivers, especially women. Due to status obligations, caregivers feel intense pressure to take care of their family members, and these processes have both structural and ideological underpinnings.[12] The ideological expectation that families should take care of their loved ones is demonstrated by a 2012 study in which the United Hospital Fund's Transitions in Care-Quality Improvement Collaborative (TC-QuIC) analyzed care transitions for family caregivers in thirty-seven hospitals, home care agencies, rehabilitation programs, and hospices. It found that of thirty-seven agencies, none had a systematic way of finding out who the actual caregiver was—only who it was assumed to be (Reinhard, Levine, and Samis 2012, 9).

The central contribution of feminist scholars in understanding caregiving labor is to show that gender often serves as an organizing principle of such labor, and that the association with love and domesticity hides the underlying work processes (Wærness 1978; Graham 1983; Ungerson 1983, 1990a). Thus, while the labor of medical professionals is visible, the labor of family caregivers seems less so—a personal matter, just what families do when one of their members is sick or in need. Activities related to caring and nurturing are often seen as the responsibility of women (Tronto 1993; Kittay 1999; Coltrane 2000; Bittman and Wajcman 2000; Bittman et al. 2003) and as something that comes "naturally" to them (Cancian and Oliker 2000; Daniels 1987). Although these activities entail large investments of time, energy, and organizational and emotional skills, they remain, for the most part, outside public discourse and invisible to society's recognition of productivity or labor processes (Daniels 1987; James 1989; DeVault 1991; Folbre 2001).

Scholars maintain that the invisibility of caring labor is rooted in the ideology of "separate spheres"—the private and public realms that became particularly prominent in the nineteenth century (Padavic and Reskin 2002).[13] Industrialization brought with it a marked change in our view of work, and relegated our measurement of productivity to economic valuations of paid work. This began a dichotomous division of labor whereby unpaid work in the "private sphere" was seen as personal and emotional, and paid work in the "public sphere" was seen as rational and productive (Coltrane and Galt 2000; Padavic and Reskin 2002).[14]

The separate-spheres construct not only fails to recognize the enormous contributions made in the private sphere, but also ideologically places "love" in the home and "labor" in paid jobs (Abel and Nelson 1990; Fisher and Tronto 1990; Glazer 1993; Cancian 2000). Angus (1994) and Glenn (2000) maintain that the relegation of emotion and the body to the private sphere denies full citizenship for caregivers, who often forego employment and retirement savings as they spend years in unpaid caregiving activity. The ideology also denies the fluidity between work and home life (Zelizer 2005), and because it contributes to cultural notions of caring as a "natural" feminine quality, serves to devalue paid care work in public sphere jobs.[15]

Feminists advocate a broader definition of work, one that takes into consideration its multifaceted nature and processes (Daniels 1987; Smith 1987; DeVault 1991, 1999; Wright 1995; Messias et al. 1997), and they have called attention to daily, unpaid work routinely performed by women as they take care of children and other dependent family members (Abel and Nelson 1990; Tronto 1993; Kittay 1999).[16] Conceptualizations of care work incorporate unpaid as well as paid labor, and their intersection between public and private worlds in a place that Stacey and Davies (1983, cited in Mayall 1993, 77) refer to as the "intermediate domain."

Past scholarship (Corbin and Strauss 1988; James 1992) demonstrates the complex and varied nature of care work. James (1992) contends that care work involves "organization," which recognizes a gendered division of labor, involves negotiating daily care, and may affect the caregiver's ability to perform paid labor; "physical labor," which includes housework and physical care work; and "emotional labor" (discussed later in this chapter). Corbin and Strauss (1988, 33–34) find that chronic illness involves complex work processes and creates an *illness trajectory*, which includes the working relationships of family, medical professionals, and the person who is chronically ill. They identify three major categories of this work: "biographical," including work related to changed identity; "illness-related," which involves medical regimens, crises, and symptom management; and "everyday-life," encompassing housework, childcare, or work in a paid job (90). Corbin and Strauss demonstrate how these types of work are interrelated and can have significant effects on the paid and unpaid work patterns and divisions of the labor of family members.

Scholars have drawn on feminist economic and philosophical literature to better synthesize and frame definitions of "care work" (Erickson and Stacey 2013; Duffy, Albelda, and Hammonds 2013). Care work scholars argue that we should analyze all care work as a single economic sector—across paid and unpaid spheres—in order to place value on its contribution to society and to inform policy (Folbre 2012a, xii; Folbre and Wright 2012; Duffy, Albelda, and Hammonds 2013, 145–46). In this vein, Nancy Folbre and Erik Olin Wright (2012, 4–5) construct three categories of care work: *interactive care*, which is often "face to face" and "hands on" and in which "concern for the well-being of the care recipient is likely to affect the quality of the services performed in interaction with that person"; *support care*, such as meal preparation, management of care, and housework, which support interactive care;[17] and *supervisory care*, which involves being "on call" and may limit other work activities.

Scant attention has been given to the study of family caregivers who are performing skilled nursing labor at home. In a study of paid caregivers in a demonstration project, Moorman and Macdonald (2012) found that caregivers who performed nursing tasks experienced more strain than those who provided personal care, and that strain was greater for those performing complex nursing tasks. Macdonald (2008) has defined "medically complex care tasks" as those that involve the operation of technological equipment, the use of sophisticated diagnostic skills, exposure to bodily fluids, and/or substantial risk to care recipients. An online study of 1,677 caregivers conducted by the AARP and the United Hospital Fund (Reinhard, Levine, and Samis 2012, 1–3) found that 46 percent of the respondents performed nursing care and that caregivers wanted more training in how to perform tasks. The authors called for more qualitative studies to better understand the interactions between caregivers and health care professionals (39). These findings support Folbre and Wright's (2012) contention that scholars must examine lived experience and qualitative interactions in care work labor processes.

Central to the exploration of lived experience is a consideration of the venue in which medical labor is carried out—the private home. Despite the paucity of research on the labor processes of caregivers who perform skilled care, we are beginning to learn more about the home context for caregivers through a diverse body of knowledge that includes the work of geographers, medical sociologists, nursing scholars, and medical practitioners.[18] Scholars have pointed out that the social meaning of "home" itself has a complex impact on identity and has multiple meanings (Cuba and Hummon 1993; Williams 2002). Culturally, "home" is endowed with feelings of privacy and security (Allan and Crow 1989; Twigg 1999; Williams 2002), but although it is often seen as a place of affection, home can also be a place of exploitation and abuse (Osmond and Thorne 1993). Moreover, home care may affect one's ideals of home life,[19] and caregivers in general may experience great isolation in their labor (Michelson and Tepperman 2003, 606; see also Boland and Sims 1996).[20] In exploring the labor of paid and unpaid workers, Glazer (1990; 1993, 178) has described a home in which skilled nursing labor takes place as a "workshop." But as opposed to a workshop or, more importantly, a hospital—a bureaucratic operation designed with medical caregiving in mind—the home is dynamic, potentially volatile, and filled with past relationship histories and unique work patterns and divisions of labor.

Toward a Synthesis of Labor Processes in Unpaid Caregiving

In this book I analyze the labor processes enacted when caregivers learn to perform skilled nursing procedures and incorporate this new work into their home life. I make the following arguments. First, it is important to realize that the nature and timing of the work, as well as the transmission of the skills, are very different from traditional family care work.[21] Skilled nursing labor requires expectations of strict schedules and objective standards that are quite different from most work performed at home—even traditional care work such as monitoring, tending, and feeding. In regard to specific skills, the interactive work process shares many features with paid care work in the public sphere. Moreover, the stakes are extremely high, and procedures that are performed inconsistently or incorrectly may have potentially devastating consequences for care recipients. Family caregivers must also learn to interact with various professionals or vendors who deliver equipment, supplies, or medicine, and who work under bureaucratic time schedules (see also Kane 1991; Twigg 2000).

Second, we must recognize the structural and ideological mechanisms at play in home health care—mechanisms that place this labor on caregivers—while also recognizing the authenticity of caregivers who want to do this type of work for those that they love, and who see themselves as capable of doing it. While there is no doubt that social structure, culture, and ideology place care within families, this book also shows that caregivers' labor is motivated by their relationships with care recipients, and that they place a priority on making their lives as normal as possible and, in many instances, keeping them out of institutions.[22] Using a labor process lens allows us to explore caregivers' feelings about the labor in the context of their relationships with care recipients, while still recognizing the tension between social structure and individual agency in the skilled labor process.[23]

Third, a significant aspect of the skilled care labor process is that caregivers must receive specific training in order to perform the technical aspects of the job. Skilled home care involves a variety of training modalities, and we do not know enough about the variations in training procedures or what they imply for the experience of unpaid skilled care work. This is unfortunate, because obtaining knowledge and gaining competency are key elements in the care labor process, and have been identified as important dimensions of caregivers' sense of well-being (Tronto 1993; Sörensen, Pinquart, and Duberstein 2002). Using a labor process lens allows us to examine the work processes that ensue and to better understand how caregivers learn to perform such procedures. In this book I show that the medical regimens of skilled nursing may be especially intense for caregivers, many of whom have little or no previous medical experience, and that caregivers are often required to learn procedures in a relatively short period of time. They cannot take advantage of prolonged and systematic on-the-job training—something that has been shown to be a valuable part of nurses' training (Davies 1995)—nor do they have the advantage of seeing multiple cases from which to gain professional expertise. Caregivers need training that is specifically tailored for their needs, backgrounds, and perceived capabilities, yet I find, through analyzing caregiver experiences, that training varies widely and is not always consistently provided.

Fourth, I find that "emotional labor" and identity (Hochschild 1983) are key dimensions of the skilled care labor process. A great deal of prior scholarship has demonstrated the complex emotional mechanisms at play in caregiving, including not only exhaustion (James 1992) and guilt (Mac Rae 1998), but also the rewards of caregiving and the importance of caregivers' relationships with care recipients and their desire to show dignity to those they care for (Abel 1991; Kittay 1999). Caregivers often go to great lengths to make sure that medical professionals understand the uniqueness of their loved ones' needs,[24] and importantly, in skilled care, they have heightened responsibility as they go from "protectors" to "performers" of care. They may worry greatly about inflicting pain or causing harm as they simultaneously perform skilled nursing procedures and offer emotional support to care recipients (see also Kohrman 1991).[25] Yet these important emotional components of the job are often not recognized by the current system, which relies on practices of standardization, places caps on nurses' visits, and does not take the particular nuances of relationships into account. The context of the home and the organization of work also affect nurses' emotional labor. They are on caregivers' and care recipients' turf and are charged with teaching very complex skills to caregivers of varying backgrounds, while working within the structural constraints that are imposed by payer sources. In order to fully understand the skilled labor process, it is critical to understand nurses' feelings regarding the labor as well as the transfer of their skills.

Finally, the current health care system, which is heavily influenced by payer sources, often boxes caregivers and care recipients into a set of choices that are far too narrow. Not everyone can perform medical procedures, and those who do have a range of unmet needs. There is great variance in caregivers' abilities, resources, health, backgrounds, and propensities to do the labor. Moreover, caregivers' ability to perform other work is tied to care recipient health, and illness may cause decreases in earning potential, the need to give up paid employment, or even poverty (Wakabayashi and Donato 2006; Glenn 2010).

In the chapters that follow, I expound on these considerations as I explore the labor processes in skilled home health care. My aim is to achieve an integrated and more complete view of the work that is involved when caregivers perform skilled medical procedures at home. I hope that all readers—including laypersons and policy makers—are enlightened by a deeper understanding of these processes.

Part I

The Work of Skilled Family Caregiving

1

The Work Caregivers Do

Learning to perform skilled nursing procedures was scary for me—an accountant/mother with no prior medical training. With detailed precision I was to deliver hospital-level antibiotics at just the right time and in precisely the right way. The drugs were always prepackaged in a seemingly comprehensive manner with cautious statements of possible side effects. Their labels listed the names of drugs I could barely pronounce, with functions I knew only at surface level. At times I wished I understood more about their chemical reactions. How exactly did they go about killing the bacteria that raged in my son's lungs? At other times I wondered if I was better off not knowing.

These stark realizations of exactly what was involved in skilled home medical labor were an awakening in what otherwise could have been construed as a fairly "normal" life. They gave me curiosity to learn about what other people were doing. What techniques were out there to master, and how difficult were they? How did other families go about this work? In our case, we experienced bouts of exhaustion as we delivered exactly what our son needed—procedures that, to me, were daunting, but that were also medically necessary.

While my husband and I learned to perform nursing procedures because our son was born with a chronic illness, caregivers come to do skilled nursing in multiple ways. Some, like us, hear a potentially devastating medical diagnosis. Others experience a sudden family tragedy, such as an accident. Some watch as loved ones undergo exacerbations of already diagnosed conditions, or make decisions that require skilled procedures in order to improve their loved ones' health or prolong their lives. The caregivers in this book represent each of these scenarios. They have learned nursing skills in order to care for loved ones who have cancer, amyotrophic lateral sclerosis (ALS), cystic fibrosis, spinal cord injury, brain injury, amputation due to diabetes, cerebral palsy, and short bowel syndrome.

In learning how to care for loved ones, caregivers like myself and my husband often have to learn procedures that are completely alien. A wife taking care of a chronically ill husband, a husband suddenly caring for his wife, aunts and uncles, grandmothers and grandfathers, parents with sick children but no medical background are now being asked to do far more than feed a family member tea and toast or chicken soup. Their tasks involve much more than giving a bed bath or changing a diaper. They involve skills that are well beyond what is generally associated with home care—tasks such as helping with activities of daily living (ADLs), like eating and dressing, or with instrumental activities of daily living (IADLs), like housework and meal preparation. As I will explain later in this chapter, caregivers are being asked to perform clinical tasks that it may take months, if not years, for a nurse to master. These include utilizing and cleaning suction tubes, feeding someone through a surgically placed gastrostomy tube (G-tube), inserting urinary catheters, administering complex regimens of IV antibiotics (all of which have potentially lethal side effects and fatal interactions), cleaning out suppurating wounds, providing drain care, and much more. Caregivers assume great amounts of risk with varying levels of resources and support. In this chapter I illuminate these physical and cognitive labor processes. I show the actual work that caregivers do.

What Caregivers Do

To describe the procedures, I begin by providing definitions of "skilled nursing care" in federally funded Medicare regulations on home care. Medicare defines skilled nursing care as "a level of care that includes services that can only be performed safely and correctly by a licensed nurse (either a registered nurse or a licensed practical nurse)" (Medicare 2011). Examples of skilled care for the Medicare home health component include "giving IV drugs, certain injections, or tube feedings; changing dressings; and teaching about prescription drugs or diabetes care" (CMS 2010b, 8).[1] The types of skilled care that caregivers administer are fundamentally determined by the particular medical situation or disease process and the decisions made by medical professionals, and they can vary greatly. Care recipients may have acute needs, postoperative needs, chronic illnesses to manage, or impaired mobility. Often, caregivers perform multiple procedures. The caregivers in this book have performed the following types of care:

TABLE 1. Types of skilled care

Skilled care procedures	Number of caregivers performing
Intravenous (IV) therapy, including intravenous antibiotics and total parenteral nutrition (TPN)	12
Feeding tubes, gastrostomy tubes, or nasogastric tubes	11
Urinary catheter care	8
Wound care and drains, pressure wounds	7
Ostomy care	2
Bowel programs	6
Tracheostomy (trach) care	6
Ventilator care	2
Operation of other machines:	
Suction catheters/machines	7
Cough assist machines	3
CPAP, bilevel pressure device (BiPAP)	4
Injections	5
Other (e.g., pump implants)	5

The duration, scope, and intensity of skilled nursing procedures vary according to the nature of the procedure and the care recipients' needs. For example, in our case, IVs were administered every six to eight hours for given periods of time when my son experienced an exacerbated lung infection. Some caregivers performed procedures multiple times a day or hour. Using a suction machine to suction mucus or saliva from a person who is having difficulty swallowing or breathing, for example, may need to be done dozens of times a day, particularly if he or she is acutely ill. Some procedures need to be performed at night, as in the case of running antibiotics or turning a person with impaired mobility. These may involve setting alarm clocks or altering sleep patterns. Changes in procedures can also occur as care recipients experience further complications or improvements in health. Some may no longer need certain procedures. Others are eventually able to perform some or all of the procedures themselves, while some, due to cognitive or physical impairments, are not.

The caregivers in this book, for the most part, did not have previous medical training.[2] Though it is beyond the scope of this book to discuss all the procedures implemented in home care, next I give a brief overview of some of the procedures that caregivers performed in order to show their importance, the details of the work, and the skill that is required.[3] Then I offer important caregiver insights, including the dilemmas they faced in grappling with this new work.

The Procedures

Intravenous therapies (IVs). IVs are used to administer medicines through the veins, and a wide range of IV therapy is now performed in homes, including IV antibiotics, total parenteral nutrition (TPN), chemotherapy, and medicines for pain control (Smith and Rothkopf 1992; Adams and Rice 2006). Medicines are generally administered through chronic intravenous central lines placed in the body. A common one for home care, and one I have worked with, is called a peripherally inserted central catheter (PICC) line, which is inserted into a vein in the arm and fed up to the superior vena cava—a large vein in the chest.[4]

As I discussed in the introduction, the formula for administering antibiotics is generally "SASH"—saline, antibiotic, saline, heparin—or a close derivative. Antibiotics are traditionally hung on IV poles and dripped, or administered through a mechanical pump. Portable pumps small enough for care recipients to carry are now used—a mother described such a pump as "about the size of a tissue box." Also available are new systems in which antibiotics come in preloaded balls, about the size and shape of a baseball, which automatically deflate and dispense medicine over time (I-Flow 2011).

In IV care, manual dexterity as well as planning, organization, and monitoring are extremely important (see Smith and Rothkopf 1992). Many IV medicines are refrigerated and taken out ahead of time before they are used (Adams and Rice 2006, 401). This means that for early morning doses, caregivers must awaken extremely early in order to set the drugs outside the refrigerator. All materials must remain uncontaminated and catheter sites must be kept sterile and monitored for signs of infection. If equipment becomes contaminated, care recipients can experience symptoms such as chills, nausea, and vomiting (Adams and Rice 2006, 396). Other complications include adverse reactions due to allergies (Smith and Rothkopf 1992, 97–99), possible blood collection or bruising at the insertion site, and circulatory overload, which occurs when too much fluid has been infused, and which can result in dizziness, coughing, or rapid pulse (Adams and Rice 2006, 394–96). Air embolism, or air in the bloodstream, can cause anxiety, shortness of breath, and even loss of consciousness—it is a medical emergency and requires that an ambulance be called (Adams and Rice 2006, 396).

Total parenteral nutrition (TPN) is a type of intravenous therapy in which nutrition is provided to individuals who are unable to effectively use their gastrointestinal tract due to a variety of conditions, such as Crohn's disease, short bowel syndrome, cancer, or ulcerative colitis (Jaudes 1991, 32; Adams and Rice 2006, 400). In TPN, nutrition is given directly into the bloodstream through a central line catheter (Jaudes 1991, 32). TPN solutions are usually dispensed over time by use of a mechanical pump (Jaudes 1991, 32; Adams and Rice 2006, 400). Blood is periodically drawn in order to monitor important indicators such as electrolyte levels and blood glucose (Jaudes 1991, 32; Adams and Rice 2006, 400). According to Adams and Rice (2006, 401), tubing must be changed every twenty-four hours, and "strict aseptic tubing standards must be met." Changing the central line dressing and the cap on the central line is a sterile procedure, which, according to one caregiver I interviewed, occurs every week. This caregiver not only performed sterile procedures but also drew up the blood work so that doctors could monitor important levels.

TPN can have serious complications. According to nursing scholars, radically changing the rate of flow can cause electrolyte imbalance, hyperglycemia, or hypoglycemia (Adams and Rice 2006, 400). Caregivers worry most about sepsis, which may occur when a bacterial or fungal infection from the catheter is spread to the bloodstream (Okun 1995, 41). According to Okun (1995, 41), other complications include fracture of the catheter and blood loss or hypoglycemia if the TPN solution accidentally becomes disconnected from the catheter.

Gastrostomy tubes (G-tubes) and nasogastric tubes (NG-tubes). Gastrostomy tubes (G-tubes) provide surgical access to the stomach for feeding or drainage. Bill, for example, described procedures he performed while maintaining a G-tube that was used for drainage when caring for his nephew. He told me he was

> maintaining . . . cleanliness for the . . . open wound [and monitoring] a G-tube that came off into a bag, that needed to be emptied if it filled. It was like . . . a collection pouch bag at the end of the . . . G-tube, . . . which had a clamp on it, and it was a matter of taking the clamp off the tube . . . [it was a] spring-release clamp and . . . so the bag came off and then could be emptied into a . . . container, milk jug, or a urine bottle. And then . . . we kept track. We kept measure . . . not an exact measure, but we kept measure about what the outflow was and then that . . . body fluid was emptied into the toilet in the bathroom. The bag then was sanitized and reattached.

When G-tubes and NG-tubes are used to place nutrition directly into the gastrointestinal tract, this process is referred to as "tube feeding" (Adams and Rice 2006, 400; Jaudes 1991, 31). Thus, when used for such purposes, it is common to refer to G-tubes and NG-tubes as "feeding tubes." While G-tubes are surgically placed into the stomach (Jaudes 1991, 31), NG-tubes are fed through the nose down into the stomach each time they are used.

Usually caregivers must deliver premixed nutritional formula into the feeding tube, but other liquids, including medicines, may also be given. Formula can be delivered through a special gravity feeding set, which is attached to an IV pole (Ahmann with revisions by Gebus 1996, 138), or an enteral (meaning "into the digestive system") feeding pump, which dispenses the formula slowly over time, may be used (Ahmann with revisions by Gebus 1996, 138; Adams and Rice 2006, 385). Several of the caregivers I interviewed set up the pumps and allowed them to run overnight. Sometimes caregivers also gave formula directly via a syringe. This is called bolus feeding and usually takes about twenty minutes or so to complete (Ahmann with revisions by Gebus 1996,138).

Both G-tubes and NG-tubes must be correctly administered and monitored, and G-tube sites must be kept clean and checked for irritation or seepage. Incorrect feeding tube procedures can cause cramping, diarrhea, bloating, vomiting, aspiration, pneumonia, and possibly even death (Ahmann with revisions by Gebus 1996, 139–42; Adams and Rice 2006, 400).

Urinary catheters. Several of the caregivers I interviewed had a great deal of experience with urinary catheters, which are used to drain urine from the bladder for people who have urinary incontinence due to a number of causes, such as bladder infections or obstructions, spinal cord injury, or illnesses such as multiple sclerosis (Houston 2006, 289; USNLM 2011e). There are three main types of urinary catheters: indwelling, external, and intermittent (Houston 2006, 291–95; USNLM 2011d). The caregivers I interviewed had experience with each of these. Indwelling catheters are "left in the bladder" (USNLM 2011d) and held there through an inflated balloon. They must be changed periodically—many protocols call for doing so every four weeks (Houston 2006, 293). A suprapubic catheter is a special kind of catheter, which also stays in place, but rather than being inserted through the urethra, it is surgically inserted into the bladder through the abdominal wall (Houston 2006, 295; USNLM 2011d). For indwelling urethral catheters, the catheter must be cleaned each day (USNLM 2011d). Suprapubic catheters, as well as the site (the opening in the stomach), need to be cleaned daily and covered with gauze (USNLM 2011d).

External catheters, also called collection devices, are primarily used in men. The most common type is a condom catheter (Houston 2006, 295; USNLM 2011d). Both indwelling and external catheters require a drainage bag, which must be emptied about every four hours or so (Houston 2006, 293) and may be strapped to the leg during the day (USNLM 2011d). Some protocols recommend periodic cleaning of the drainage bag (USNLM 2011d).

Intermittent catheters are inserted to drain the bladder and are taken out once the flow of urine has stopped (USNLM 2011d). These are sometimes called "in and out" catheters because the individual is "catheter free" until it is time to drain the bladder (AUAF 2010). Some caregivers who practiced in-and-out catheterization worried that they might hurt the care recipient when inserting the catheter.

Proper urinary catheterization is important to ensure the vital kidney function of care recipients. One of the biggest complications caregivers identified with catheterization was the risk of urinary tract infections (UTIs) (see also Houston 2006, 292). To decrease this risk, hand washing and proper care of the catheter are essential. There is also a risk of obstruction, leakage (due to obstruction or bladder spasms), blocked drainage (due to the catheter becoming encrusted with debris), and skin breakdown (292).

Wound care. Wound care may be necessary for care recipients with acute wounds, resulting from surgical incisions or trauma, or chronic wounds, which may result from underlying disease processes such as vascular insufficiency or diabetes (Rice, Wiersema-Bryant, and Bangert 2006, 240). One type of chronic wound, called pressure ulcers (or bedsores), occurs when there is "excessive, unrelieved pressure or from external forces such as shearing or friction" (243). Patients who are immobile and lie in one position for a long time are especially at risk. Several caregivers had loved ones who were susceptible to bedsores, and they often had to get up in the middle of the night to reposition or turn them. Pressure-reduction devices such as trapeze bars or side rails on beds can help with turning or moving, and pressure-relief devices such as air flotation beds may also be used (252–54). One mother told me that even though they have an air mattress, she still gets up "at least once a night" to "flip" her son. "Basically," she said, "it's a safety thing for me, you know, stop his skin from breaking down even more."

Characteristics of the wound, such as its type, depth, and location, all affect how care is performed. Cleanliness, including hand washing and use of gloves if prescribed, and monitoring for changes in size, color, or drainage, are extremely important (Rice, Wiersema-Bryant, and Bangert 2006, 247). In some cases, sterile dressings may need to be applied frequently. Some wounds may need to be irrigated or surgically debrided, which involves surgically removing nonviable tissue (252).

One type of wound care—"wet to dry" dressing changes—involves placing wet gauze dressing into a wound, and allowing the dressing to dry out so that wound drainage and dead tissue adhere to it. The old dressing is then pulled out and replaced with a new dressing (USNLM 2011e).

Annette described this kind of postsurgery wound care, which she performed for her mother:

> I had to learn how to take the dressing, and put on the gloves, and everything had to be sterile. And it had to be, I think it was called wet to dry; it had to have the wet dressing inside so it was almost like a Vaseline-covered type of bandage. . . . We used a tube [of saline] each time that we did it, and we would . . . squirt it inside, and then clean it out. You know, soak it up with the gauze. Take the gauze out. Then we would take the Vaseline-soaked bandage and put it down in . . . and we'd have to cut a strip so it matched whatever size the wound was, and keep cutting down, as the wound healed, and it wasn't so big anymore. And then we would cover that with gauze. . . . We would tape over [the] top to hold it all in.

Rita worked with a wound VAC (vacuum-assisted closure), a vacuum that uses negative pressure to clean out wound drainage. This machine usually has a pump and a sponge that attaches to an open wound and "essentially converts an open wound into a controlled closed wound" (Rice, Wiersema-Bryant, and Bangert 2006, 252). According to Rita, the tricky part of using a wound VAC was monitoring to make sure the suction is maintained. She experienced several problems with the pump and had to call for and receive assistance from the home health agency. "The bag part of it," she said, "it's like anything mechanical, you know, at the worst time it will get a leak and then it makes a horrible noise and you're trying to do everything to try to get it resealed and stuff, and that's where I would try to help, doing those kind of things. And then we'd have to call the poor home health nurses and then they'd have to come at various and sundry times. . . . You can't have any leak . . . because then you lose the suction. . . . It's gotta be airtight."

Ostomy. When an operation is performed to create a new opening (called a stoma) in the abdomen, the surgery is called an ostomy (USNLM 2018). There are many different kinds of ostomies, and their names depend on the location of the surgery. For example, in percutaneous (through-the-skin) nephrostomy, a catheter is placed through the skin into the kidney in order to drain the kidney (USNLM 2011b). In colostomy, the rectum and anus are bypassed, and the colon is attached to the new stoma (USNLM 2018). An ostomy bag is connected to the stoma and is worn outside the body to collect waste.

Ostomy care depends on the type of procedure performed and the body organs involved. Here a caregiver described a nephrostomy:

> Okay, a nephrostomy is a colostomy except it's not in the colon. It's an ostomy that is in your kidney. . . . And there's a drain tube that goes into the kidney and it picks up the urine and it comes out. And then she [the caregiver's wife] wore a leg bag. . . . I had to change the bag. And then there was a connecting tube between the nephrostomy tube and the bag. . . . And there's also a support bandage that fits on the body to hold that tube so it doesn't go in and out, in and out. . . . And so that has to be changed every two weeks.

Caregivers who take care of colostomies must learn how to change the ostomy pouch to dispose of body waste. This involves careful cleaning of their hands and the skin around the stoma, checking the stoma site, measuring the stoma, reattaching a new pouch, and checking for signs of infection (USNLM 2011a).

Bowel management programs. Caregivers may also perform bowel management programs for those who have suffered nerve or neurological damage due to spinal cord injury, or who have other illnesses or injuries. The program is used to keep the care recipient on an effective schedule and may include diet changes and various bowel routines (USNLM 2019). A technique that is often used is digital stimulation, which involves "circular motion with the index finger in the rectum" so that the person can defecate (NRSCIS 2011). Suppositories or enemas may also be used. Bowel programs generally take about thirty to sixty minutes to perform and are tailored to the specific needs and preferences of the individual (NRSCIS 2011).

Respiratory procedures. For care recipients who have respiratory compromise due to a variety of reasons such as brain injury, ALS, or spinal cord injury, a suction machine is often used to help clear secretions out of the airways. Essentially, a catheter is connected to the suction machine and then inserted gently into the back of the throat or nose (Ahmann with revisions by Page 1996, 177–78). It is important to be gentle due to the potential for tissue destruction and bleeding (177). Catheters must be cleaned between each pass (177). Secretions are pulled into a suction canister, which, along with the tubing, must be cleaned daily (Rice 2006b, 229). In case of a power outage or electrical failure, a manual mouth-suction device must be available in the home (Ahmann with revisions by Page 1996, 180).

A tracheostomy, a type of stoma, is an opening in the throat that allows a person to breathe when the airway has been compromised; the tracheostomy tube serves as an "artificial airway" (Rice 2006b, 219). In order to take care of a tracheostomy, a person must know how to suction secretions, how to remove and insert the tracheostomy tube, and how to follow the correct emergency procedures if there are problems with insertion or the care recipient has difficulty breathing (Driscoll 1996, 221–25). Suctioning should be performed carefully, and the suctioning catheter should be inserted just below the tip of the artificial airway (Driscoll 1996, 224; Rice 2006b, 229). When I visited with Randy, who provided care for his son, he told me that catheters are marked so that the caregiver can follow the numbers and know how far in to place it when suctioning: "Well . . . on the catheters they got numbers on there. . . . Your trach is only like [at] the six or something. . . . He's got numbers on it . . . on the side there. And it's . . . six inch to seven inch to eight inch to nine and so forth."

Some nursing literature recommends changing tracheostomy tubes at least once a week for infants and children and once a month for adults (Driscoll 1996, 224; Rice 2006b, 228). Changing tracheostomy tubes can cause anxiety for care recipients and caregivers alike. A device called an obturator is used to insert the outer cannula (tube that holds the stoma open) of the tracheostomy tube and must be removed very quickly because it temporarily occludes the airway (Rice 2006b, 220). It is also important for caregivers to clean the stoma daily and to apply a clean, "absorbent, lint-free" dressing around it (229). Stomas should be inspected to make sure there is no redness or infection (229).

Clearly, providing tracheostomy care is a complex and risky undertaking. Phoebe described taking care of a trach for her son:

> Well they had a plug over it, which was basically a voice box. . . . It blocked the air so he could talk. . . . We had to take that off and shove a tube, probably a six-inch tube, down in there, and cover a hole and let it suck it out as we moved it around to knock some other stuff loose . . . and then pull it back out. And the mucus and stuff was always stuck to the outside of the tube and you always had to have gloves on of course, 'cause you didn't want to put an infection directly *in* there. . . . It went into a machine that had a

canister that you had to clean the canister out and it always had to be carried with you. It was always with you. When we left the hospital they said there's three things that you have to have with you at all times. The suction bag, which [is] very heavy, an Ambu bag, which is basically a rescuer [you] put . . . either over their mouth or over their trach and then they can breathe . . . and . . . saline, which you could put down in there and break up the stuff in his chest.

Because obstruction of the airway is a life-threatening condition, caregivers must be well versed in emergency procedures and have supplies readily available (Driscoll 1996, 223). Nursing scholars recommend keeping extra tracheostomy tubes on hand, including tubes that are one size smaller, in case the regular tracheostomy tube cannot be inserted (Driscoll 1996, 223; Rice 2006b, 228). If the smaller tube cannot be inserted for an infant, Driscoll (1996, 225) recommends that the "suction catheter . . . be placed in the stoma, secretions removed, and breaths given through the catheter." CPR may need to be used and emergency personnel called. If the tube cannot be properly inserted for an adult, Rice (2006b, 228) recommends that the caregiver use her or his hand to make a tight seal over the stoma and apply manual ventilation with an Ambu bag (a balloon-like apparatus that blows air into the lungs) and face mask until emergency backup arrives. Unfortunately, not all emergency rescue squads have experience with trachs (Driscoll 1996, 225). I learned this from a few of the caregivers I spoke with. One had to suction a trach even after an emergency squad was called because the EMTs did not know how to perform the procedures.

If those receiving care need assistance in order to breathe, they will be attached to a mechanical ventilator that "moves air into the lungs" (Ahmann with revisions by Jerome-Ebel 1996, 236). Today, positive-pressure ventilators are most often used; these push air directly into the lungs through either a face/nose mask or a tracheostomy tube (Ahmann with revisions by Jerome-Ebel 1996, 237; Okun 1995, 36). Though there are different types of positive-pressure ventilators, often volume-controlled ventilators—which deliver breaths based on a preset volume—are used for home care (Ahmann with revisions by Jerome-Ebel 1996, 237; Rice 2006b, 218, 231). Portable lightweight models are battery operated and are small enough for travel or for attachment to a wheelchair (Okun 1995, 36; Rice 2006b, 218). A mother explained that this model involved making sure that the settings were right, the tubes were clean. You . . . always had to have saline, like for moisture, . . . a saline bag. . . . He had a little laptop; well, it's called a laptop ventilator. And it hung on the back of his chair. You just kinda make sure it always stayed connected and always stayed charged up. . . . You can have like a huge battery. It runs probably [a] couple of days. It's an external battery that is actually put on the wheelchair. . . . You can just hook it into the wheelchair.

Positive-pressure ventilators are set up so that alarms sound if the person becomes disconnected, or if there is an obstruction between the machine and the person's lungs (Okun 1995, 36). Some people who are on ventilators require additional oxygen, but others do not (219).

Obviously, there is a great deal of responsibility and time commitment for the caregiver who is caring for a ventilator-dependent person. Serious complications, including death, can occur due to machine failure or airway obstruction (Okun 1995, 38). Complete knowledge of the ventilator machine and its operation is required, and family members need to be prepared in case of emergency. They need to understand the signs of respiratory distress or failure, and they should know CPR (Ahmann with revisions by Jerome-Ebel 1996, 238). If a person requires continuous ventilation, a backup system must be in place in the home, including a self-inflating manual ventilator (Ambu bag); an identical second ventilator is also often used (Rice 2006b, 220). Area emergency personnel need to be alerted, as do telephone and utility companies, so families can be on a priority basis if there is a power outage (Ahmann with revisions by Jerome-Ebel 1996, 238). One caregiver told me that her home had to be inspected to make sure there were proper power systems in place.

Noncontinuous ventilator support for people who do not have a tracheostomy can sometimes be achieved by use of a continuous positive airway pressure (CPAP) machine or through a bilevel pressure device (often referred to as a BiPAP) (Rice 2006b, 219). Individuals who have sleep apnea or neuromuscular dysfunction may use these machines (219). Typically a mask is worn, which connects to the machine by tubing. One caregiver found the BiPAP awkward and difficult to operate, and said the "alarm wouldn't stop going off at night."

Individuals who are paralyzed or who have trouble generating a cough may also need a cough assist machine to help clear lung secretions.

Individuals are usually connected to the machine by tubing and a mask, and when they breathe in, the machine delivers air to the lungs, then creates a sucking force during exhale (UW Health 2010). A caregiver who uses a cough assist machine for her son described it as "like a vacuum cleaner. . . . It forces air in and sucks it out so it helps suck out the mucus . . . because he can't cough. . . . He has no cough muscles."

Other procedures. Caregivers also perform many other procedures, including taking vital signs, watching for signs and symptoms, giving injections, monitoring seizures, dispensing medication, and drawing blood. They perform procedures associated with respiratory or physical therapy, such as administering aerosolized breathing treatments and chest physical therapy, performing physical therapy or range-of-motion exercises, and—for care recipients with mobility issues—transporting, lifting, or using machinery such as a Hoyer lift for such purposes. Nine caregivers learned transport techniques and five used Hoyer lifts or other electric lifts. Caregivers also assist with pump implants, which continually deliver medication through implanted catheters. For example, some pumps deliver insulin for diabetes control (ADA 2011), while others deliver medicine to reduce muscle spasticity caused by brain or nerve damage (USNLM 2011c).

Caregiver Insights and Dilemmas in Providing Skilled Care

Caregivers revealed many important insights about the work they did. In general, many of the medical procedures are not only difficult to master but also cause trepidation because of the possible complications that can result if the caregiver makes a mistake.[5] Several caregivers who gave IVs said they worried about contaminating the IV site or shooting air in the line. Bridget indicated that she got only a quick lesson in the administration of IV antibiotics and that this exacerbated her anxiety about the possible consequences of performing the procedures incorrectly: "You gotta show me, and you gotta show me more than once. I mean I gotta do it two or three times, you know, before—and then I'm never sure. Especially with this type thing, you know? Because you're dealing with somebody's health. . . . That was my biggest worry."

In hospitals, problems with medication administration are a leading cause of death, and so are infections that occur when a wound is not correctly dressed or an IV carefully accessed. Yet family caregivers are asked to do these activities on a routine basis—over a period of months or even years.

Moreover, as Bridget's comment reveals, the fear of making mistakes adds significant worry because caregivers know that the procedures have serious implications for the health of their loved ones (see also Kohrman 1991). Annette, who performed "wet to dry" wound care for her mother, was extremely nervous the first time she did the procedure on her own because she was afraid she would hurt her mother: "I told Mom I was shaking. And she said, 'Just don't drop the scissors in there.' [*Chuckles.*] And so, I was afraid I was going to hurt her because I couldn't tell how hard to push and I didn't want to push because she would moan and groan anyway, the way it was. Because it just . . . was so tender." Annette thus had to control her own fears as she simultaneously worked through the procedure with her mother in order to perform the vital wound care tasks that were needed.

The worry about complications is well founded, as they can have deleterious consequences. Meredith, who performs TPN, said that sepsis is her main fear and that she must be diligent—not only to make sure that everything is sterile, but also to monitor for any signs of infection. She told me, "The stress of it is, the central line can kill him. If he gets sepsis . . . any episode can kill him."

Coupled with issues of anxiety and fear of causing harm to the care recipient are issues of manual dexterity and "getting the feel" of the procedures. Elle, who had to push a large 30 cc syringe, told me that it was hard to "have my thumb up there ready" and still guide it properly, and according to Cheryl, "getting the feel" of placing an NG-tube can be very tricky. She told me,

> It took me a while to figure out. I mean she [the home health nurse] had the patience of a saint.'Cause when you start to inch the tube in the nose, it . . . meets a significant amount of resistance. And . . . even though [my child's] swallowing, . . . you have to push straight back. I always thought you kind of would like have to curve it . . . but it's a straight-back motion. Took me a while to get . . . how that was. . . . But she had patience and so I got it past that rough spot. [My child's] swallowing the water. The tube goes all the way down. It's marked . . . on the tube. So when you get that little marked tube to the edge of her nose, you know you've gone far enough.

For caregivers like Cheryl, this new work is not only strange but even counterintuitive. Not only did she have to get past her initial fears, but she had to learn to get the tube past the point of resistance. She said she also had to make sure the procedure was performed quickly in order to reduce her child's discomfort: "It very quickly goes through and you just keep shoving—trying to do this kind of motion . . . shove-shove-shove-shove. . . . You wanna do this fast. . . . You want to . . . get it over with. . . . So you keep pushing until you get to that mark . . . you know, by the edge of her nose? . . . Then . . . you use Tegaderm and you tape it to her face."

Securing the NG-tube, however, is not the final step of the procedure, as caregivers must then check for proper placement. This is an important step because aspiration can occur if tubes are improperly placed into the lungs rather than the stomach (Ahmann with revisions by Gebus 1996, 141). One way to check is to position a stethoscope over the stomach and quickly inject a small amount of air into the tube, then listen for a popping sound (141).

Cheryl: Then the next step is to know—did you put it down the esophagus or the trachea? . . . So what you do then is you put on a stethoscope . . . and you lay the stethoscope on the stomach. . . . And then you shoot air into the tube and if it's in the stomach it's gonna go, "Blumb-blumb, blumb-blumb." You'll hear it through the stethoscope because you're mixing the stomach contents with the air.
Interviewer: So you hear the noise if it's in the stomach?
Cheryl: [*Nods.*]
Interviewer: Okay.
Cheryl: If you don't hear anything, that's not good. I've never put it down the trachea. I've never . . . I don't know if she would have . . . would choke more, you know? But every single time the tube is placed it must be . . . confirmed with the stethoscope and the pushing of the air. Every time.

As shown in this example, precision and timing are essential in performing skilled nursing tasks. When Morgan described suctioning for her husband, she likewise stated that timing was a key element. If she didn't do the procedure for long enough, there was the danger of not clearing secretions so he could breathe, yet, as she explained, "You can only hold it so long, and suck so long because it cuts off their oxygen while you're doing it. I always thought, 'I'm gonna kill him.'"

Some caregivers also felt they needed help for some procedures. In describing in-and-out (or "straight," as she called it) catheterizations for her husband, Morgan was extremely concerned about the correct insertion and cleanliness of the catheter. As her comment illustrates, caregivers sometimes wish for an extra pair of hands. "You have a kit that's all sterile," she said, "so you have to go through making a sterile field, you know, opening it . . . right. You needed an assistant, which was hard, 'cause I didn't always have one."

Indeed, in my personal experience, I often felt there were not as many hands as I needed. For example, I found it hard to pull the cap off a syringe of saline while holding the IV catheter correctly so as not to contaminate it. I sometimes pulled the cap off with my teeth because I had seen a home health nurse do that once.

Not only do caregivers have to overcome fear, get the feel of procedures, and make sure they are done correctly, but they also have to get past the personal discomfort they may have regarding the intimate nature of the work they are asked to do. Sociologists have referred to body work as work that is "performed on behalf of or directly on other peoples' [*sic*] bodies" (Gimlin 2007, 358).[6] Twigg and colleagues (2011, 172) note that body work is "often ambivalent work that may violate the norms of the management of the body, particularly in terms of touch, smell or sight." Scholars maintain that such work is generally seen as the responsibility of women, and they have focused on the power dynamics at play—both between patients and medical professionals and among providers themselves (Gimlin 2007, 358). With regard to medical professionals, Twigg (2000, 390) makes the point that those with higher status engage in distancing techniques, and that as nurses move up in their careers, "they move away from the basic bodywork of bedpans and sponge baths towards high-tech, skilled interventions; progressing from dirty work on bodies to clean work on machines."

Home care introduces a context in which paid professionals, family caregivers, and care recipients must negotiate and give meaning to the body work that must be performed (England and Dyck 2011). In this regard, it is notable that unpaid caregivers do not have formal job status or job hierarchies. Their work often includes mundane, frequently "messy" and "dirty" work related to the human bodies of those with whom they have a personal relationship, as well as work that involves high-tech equipment and sterile procedures. A nurse noted this tension when she said that one obstacle in home care is that for body areas considered private, "caregivers can't handle seeing that person in that state," and that care recipients may not want their family members to give them this kind of care.

Indeed, some caregivers were placed into positions they had never imagined being in, such as diapering adult loved ones, performing catheterizations, or implementing bowel routines like inserting suppositories or manually stimulating the rectum. Several confided that this was not an easy process for them, but they knew it was necessary for their loved one's health, and so they did it. Caregivers also had to deal with unwelcome and unpleasant sights and smells, referring to some things as "gross" or "yucky." Wound tissue smelled "just like a dead animal," a caregiver told me.

Others were squeamish about peering into body cavities, cleaning up body fluids, or tending to wounds. The fact that care recipients are loved ones no doubt affects the caregivers' reaction. Bill recounted the first time the doctor explained the procedures for taking care of his nephew's wound and G-tube: "I can recall so vividly the doctor with his . . . plastic gloves on, inserting his fingers into the body cavity there . . . and I'm seeing this and I'm, yes, conjuring up the thought . . . 'What am I getting myself into?' And [*sighs heavily*] . . . that thought will never leave me."

Of course, reactions to the body and feelings about carrying out medical labor vary among individuals. Paul said he was able to perform his wife's wound care and other medical procedures without letting his feelings about the body bother him because he knew it was simply something that needed to be done: "I'm an engineer at heart. . . . And so . . . well it's a matter-of-fact thing. You know? It . . . wasn't an issue of being afraid to do it. It was just I knew what to do—and we do it." Several caregivers, however, candidly confessed that performing skilled nursing care was very difficult and that they constantly struggled with their new work. No matter what their response or readiness for this, seeing loved ones in pain, or having to dress their wounds, was a reality many caregivers had to face. A wife told me, "It's just something that you don't get over real fast. . . . It's just something you never thought you'd see. . . . It was an emotional time, I'll tell you that."

As demonstrated, the labor that caregivers perform involves risk, manual dexterity, knowledge, and precision. It is very intense work that carries high stakes and can cause anxiety and emotion management for caregivers who are implementing it (see chapter 5 for a discussion of emotion work). The kinds of procedures I described above are things that in hospitals and other health care settings are always done by professional caregivers—that is, registered nurses—who are licensed and who belong to professional organizations. Yet today's increasingly complex requirements to become a nurse—including having sophisticated knowledge, mastering new technologies, and achieving professional credentials (see NCSBN 2011a, 2011b)—parallel, somewhat ironically, the transfer of nursing skills back home to caregivers—caregivers who may have little or no previous medical training.

2

On-the-Job Training

I first learned to do skilled care work from home health nurses on the afternoon my son was discharged from the hospital. I was shocked by how much I had to learn, and how quickly. The tasks themselves seemed far beyond me. It was hard to grasp the fact that I would be doing this—today, right now, in my home—and that a mistake could injure my son.

The nurses gave me a few hours of instruction and let me know I would be on my own the very first night. I wondered at the time how common this was, and so when I later conducted interviews with caregivers, I let them speak openly about how they learned to do skilled care. I was struck by the fact that they had learned to do skilled nursing in multiple ways. Some had learned a great deal before discharge. Others, like me, had learned very little.

The structure of the U.S. health care system itself may be partly to blame for these variances.[1] Rather than a seamless continuum of care, critics describe the various institutional actors as stand-alone "silos" that are often unconnected to each other. Hospitals have their own ways of handling patient communication and caregiver training, and relationships between hospitals, physicians, and home health agencies vary, and often stem from past arrangements and affiliations. This was a major point made by many home health nurses I interviewed when they spoke of the difficulties in coordinating care. Some groups of doctors or providers were easier to work with than others. They offered more support and respect for home health nurses' assessments and provided better channels of communication.

Homecoming and Nurses' Teaching Strategies

When I talked with home health nurses about how they teach, it was evident that they develop strategies based on caregivers' and care recipients' readiness and different levels of knowledge. One of the first things they say they do in making initial contact is to find out what the expectations are, and manage them. According to Jamie, "I always start out asking them what they know already. . . . 'Have you ever seen this before? You ever heard of this? Do you understand the diagnosis and why this caused that?' . . . Find out what knowledge they already have . . . and then just build it up from there." Many nurses say that because they know caregivers can be overwhelmed, they prefer to "start with the basics" or teach "a little bit at a time." Ruth told me, "I try to . . . limit the amount of information I give them all at one time . . . because . . . who can comprehend all that? You know? You're overwhelmed with just bringing your loved one home and your responsibility of needing to . . . prepare meals and go to the grocery and help with their medication."

Another strategy nurses say they use, especially if someone is hesitant or has anxiety, is to give emotional reassurance, including "lots of praise," positive reinforcement, and encouragement. (See chapter 6 for a discussion of emotional labor.) As Les said, "You have to encourage them. You have to empower them." Nurses say they have told caregivers, "You did a fine job doing that," "Give yourself a pat on the back," "Boy—this sure looks better," "You *can* do this. I *know* you can do this and you *will* do this. *We* will do this and then *you* will do this." One nurse said she sometimes gives hugs. Nurses also said they try to correct in a positive way. One nurse stated that it is important to "focus on the things they're struggling with without making them feel incompetent." Some nurses say they also have reassured caregivers that they would not hurt their loved ones. Dana told a woman who was going to learn how to give an IV, and who was "in a state of panic" on the phone, "Anything that I'm going to bring with me will not harm the patient because I won't *let* it happen."

In terms of hands-on work, all nurses say that the general process is to demonstrate to the caregiver and/or care recipient exactly what they are to do, allow them to watch and ask questions, and then observe a return demonstration. Nurses describe demonstrating as "walking through" the steps or "talking through" the procedures as they are doing them. In a return demonstration, caregivers or care recipients must show the nurse that they can perform all the procedures on their own. From talking with caregivers, this method was generally employed; however, a few times it was not, as in the case of discharge delays.

It is evident from listening to both nurses and caregivers that there is a great deal of variability in how home health nurses convey information. While some of this may be due to agency policies or norms, nurses have different teaching philosophies and styles and are often given much lee-way as to how they transmit information. Six nurses say they write every-thing down in a step-by-step protocol for the caregiver, and three others say that step-by-step instructions for common procedures are prewritten by their agencies. Others say that whether they write down instructions, or whether they have caregivers repeat the protocols before allowing them to perform the procedures themselves, depends on the situation. Nurses also report drawing pictures and diagrams, sometimes as a supplement to written procedures, and commonly as a guide for those who cannot read or have trouble reading the English language.

Nurses observe that some caregivers take their own notes, while others do not. Seven caregivers in this study said they took notes or wrote down instructions on the correct way to do the procedures. This appeared to be a personal choice in most cases; as one caregiver said, "I'm a writer-downer." Some of the difference in methods, however, was due to the teaching strategies employed by home health nurses. For example, in one case, a caregiver was not given a written protocol on IVs prior to arriving home, but the home health nurse wrote down step-by-step instructions for her. The caregiver believed these instructions to be extremely helpful and said she referred to them on multiple occasions.

Nurses say a key feature of their job is building rapport, gaining trust, and establishing common ground. They emphasize the common goal of both caregivers and nurses—to help the care recipient maintain health, heal, or gain more independence. Some nurses believe that by talking about this objective, caregivers can better picture the end result and realize why their work is important. Regarding a foot wound, Chloe gave this example: "Wouldn't you like to see them up and walking around again? . . . We gotta get this foot better."

In establishing common goals, a significant strategy nurses use is to reduce their own status of "medical expert" when interacting with families.[2] A nurse explained, "You don't want them to feel like you're up here and they're down here . . . We're all on the same field at the same level, trying to do the same goal." Nurses recognize that caregivers may be unfamiliar with medical language, and say they are careful to "not talk over their heads" or to "bring it down to their level." Said Dana, "I don't want to go in and, because I got a degree in nursing, sit there and talk all this medical stuff, and they're looking at ya, and you know . . . their head's sideways and they say 'Uh-huh.' And you turn around and walk out and they don't have a clue what you tried to explain to 'em." In attempting to speak a common language, Karen explained, "I'll call it an IV tubing, but then when they look at me and they call it a hose . . . from now on, we call it a hose, and I'll say, 'The IV tubing, or a hose as you call it.'" One nurse gave the example of teaching an elderly woman who had baked all her life that giving an IV has some similarities to the baking process: "'Here's the supplies that we need to do the infusion,' as compared to 'Here's the supplies we need to bake a cake.' . . . You have to get all your equipment out, you gotta get your bowls and your mixers. . . . Now you need your ingredients. . . .' Sometimes you have to break it down to—how they can understand."

Nurses believe that skills can be taught quite well to those with limited formal education. They also clearly stated that a person's ability to learn was not based on the individual's socioeconomic status. Jamie told me, "I can take somebody with a PhD that can't grasp what I'm trying to tell her, but somebody that didn't graduate high school can."

While knowing nurses' strategies is foundational in understanding the interactional transfer of their skills to caregivers, the structural limitations imposed by payer sources also shape their interactions (see chapter 3). For example, while nurses generally prefer to teach slowly, they are sometimes constrained by how many visits payer sources allow. Nurses are very conscientious of this, and try to do the teaching in the first few visits, when caregivers need more help and care recipients are especially vulnerable to hospital readmission. Some of the nurses called this strategy "frontloading visits."

Structural limitations may also mean that nurses are forced to change the way they teach; for example, they may have caregivers do more work sooner than the nurses would prefer. One nurse said that it's frustrating when insurance is "not gonna pay for the nurse to come." She told me, "Maybe we're just getting two visits to go out and teach somebody and that's it. So . . . then . . . you're forcing them to *have* to learn." Another nurse was upset because she did not feel she was granted adequate time to teach a patient who needed IV care, additional education, and blood draws. The patient was also single and did not have a caregiver available. In explaining her frustration with the limitations, she said, "It's just a lot . . . for being . . . single. You rig up a contraption that can hold the PICC [peripherally inserted central catheter] line still so you can screw it into your own arm. I mean, that's hard."

Virtually all nurses said they reassure caregivers and care recipients that they should call if they have any questions or if the care recipient has signs or symptoms of a problem. As Josephine said regarding a wound, "Watch for infection, redness, swelling, drainage." Most of them said their agencies have a twenty-four-hour phone number. One nurse told me she makes sure to convey to her patients that "there's always somebody available to talk. . . . If you have any questions, call us. If you want to call us while you're doing the dressing, then we can walk you through it, and that's fine."

While caregivers I interviewed said they were comforted because they knew they could always call, most said they tried to figure things out on their own and called only if they felt it was absolutely necessary. Many discussed ways in which they actively problem solved on their own (see chapter 4). Several described doing substantial research, including finding online sources, to try to supplement their knowledge. Moreover, as Albert (1990) and Corbin and Strauss (1990) found in their work on the elderly and those with chronic illnesses, respectively, there is a great amount of trial and error in home care experiences. This is also the case with specific skilled procedures. A caregiver who was performing suctioning for her son told me, "We learned that . . . what works for one person doesn't necessarily work for the next. . . . So, we just sort of learned what the best method was for him through trial and error." Some caregivers also noticed that medical professionals seemed to perform procedures differently, and so they came up with their own methods. When Bridget learned to bandage her husband's leg, she devised her own technique based on her observations and consultations with her husband.[3] Bridget's husband later told me, "She could do it better than they did."

How Do They Learn?

The fragmented nature of the system means that caregivers may experience vast differences in communication processes and in the training they receive. In 2002, a national telephone survey of caregivers found that although 43 percent were responsible for nursing skills such as bandaging and wound care, the operation of pumps or machines, or medication administration (of which one-sixth was non-oral), about 33 percent said they received no instruction on dressing and bandaging or the use of equipment, and 18 percent received no instruction on medication administration (Donelan et al. 2002, 227). As noted in the introduction of this book, a 2012 online study found that caregivers wanted more training in how to perform nursing tasks (Reinhard, Levine, and Samis 2012, 1–3). A 2015 quantitative online interview study of 1,248 caregivers of adults, conducted by the National Alliance for Caregiving and the AARP Public Policy Institute, found that although 57 percent assisted with nursing tasks, 42 percent reported that they were doing so without having received any preparation or training (NAC and AARP 2015, 17).

The caregivers in this book primarily had loved ones who were discharged from hospitals or rehabilitation facilities, although a few were discharged from clinics or doctors' offices. Many had been in multiple care settings. There was wide variability in the training received. Caregivers with loved ones in rehabilitation facilities received intense practice over multiple days, while other caregivers received only some or very little training prior to discharge. While some of this variability was dictated by the particular medical condition, I also found that training processes were affected by differences in institutional practices as well as by the actions of institutional personnel. For example, caregivers who had loved ones with similar medical conditions had different experiences across institutions. Ava, whose husband had cancer surgery, was shown very little about how to irrigate his wound in the hospital and was not assigned home health care. Paul, whose wife had cancer surgery, was shown by medical personnel how to take care of the wound, was assigned home health care, and was even given the doctor's cell phone number in case he had questions. There were also cases where caregivers identified particular personnel who, possibly due to time-constraint pressures, did not do what they considered a thorough job of teaching.

The particular institutional experiences, including communication processes, prior to discharge greatly shape caregivers' reactions to the labor and their feelings about their own competency right off the bat. Next I explore caregivers' training experiences prior to discharge from hospitals and other institutions.

Caregivers Who Received Prolonged Training in Rehabilitation Facilities and Hospitals

Several caregivers received prolonged training in rehabilitation facilities or hospitals, which were located in five different states in the midwestern, eastern, and southern regions of the U.S. Generally, in these cases, care recipients had suffered critical injuries such as spinal cord or brain injuries and were admitted for long periods of time, usually at least two to three months. In most instances, at least two caregivers were required to learn the procedures. A home health nurse told me about a mother and son who had brought the woman's husband home from one of these facilities. Although she had to train them on an IV he needed, she said, "they came home pretty much knowing his trach care and his ventilator [care]."

Although these caregivers' stories varied with respect to their own perceptions and experiences, most of the caregivers noted how the training they received increased their feelings of competency. This appeared to be due not only to the quality and extent of the training, but also to the gradual nature in which it was introduced. According to Faye,

> When you first get there, they kinda do . . . everything. And then as . . . his health became . . . pretty much stable, they would gradually introduce me

to learn how to suction him, learn how to use a cough assist machine. . . .
They have like overhead lifts. . . . They would do it and they'd say, "Here,
try this." And they'd always be there with me . . . to make sure I knew how
to do everything. And it just was . . . *everything*—from giving him a bath,
to washing his hair, to . . . taking care of his tracheostomy. So it started
with them doing it and then as I felt better . . . a little bit more relaxed,
that's when they pretty much encourage you to do all hands on so that you
know how to do everything when you get home. . . . I could do as little as
I wanted or as much as I wanted. But by the time I left there, I knew how
to do everything.

A significant feature of this training involved spending the night alone
with the care recipient and performing all procedures before discharge—
what some of the nurses referred to as "transitional care." This seemed to
resonate with caregivers, and they believed this process to be a powerful
evaluation of their ability to perform the job. Faye described the program
she was in as a "test run." It wasn't, she said, "like you're locked in there
or anything—but unless there was an emergency, there was *no* nurse that
would come in and help you." Simon told me that even though he and his
wife performed all the procedures for their son in the hospital, they knew
that hospital staff members were only minutes away if they needed them:
"They told us from the get-go . . . if you're not comfortable, you can push
this button and we'll come in and help you. But we're not gonna let you
take him home until you're *ready* to take care of him." Some caregivers
noted that their experience in rehab also taught them how to perform vigilant monitoring. Connor said, "They taught us over there not just to do
the physical cathing of someone or helping them in the shower . . . but to
look at the overall perspective. 'Are you sure you took some of this medicine? . . . Be very observant because things can happen very quickly. . . .
You look at the whole system. . . . You look for bedsores . . . every day.
Don't let it go a day.' "

Although these caregivers believed they had received very good or even
excellent training, many still said they were scared or anxious when they
arrived home and had to perform the procedures for the first time completely on their own. Moreover, the home experience itself varied for caregivers. Some still had to interact more directly with home care nurses as
they learned to manipulate new pumps or equipment. Isabelle and Randy,
whose infant son had a brain injury, were shown how to suction his trach

and do tube feedings during their one-month hospital stay, but still said they depended greatly on home health nurses to educate them on trach care and other procedures.

Other caregivers said that home health nurses came more or less to perform vitals and check on them. In fact, some of these caregivers felt they had more knowledge of how to treat the care recipient than did some local home health nurses. A mother who learned how to take care of her son—who had a tracheostomy, and was on a ventilator—in a rehab facility in a larger city away from her home state said that once they arrived home, home health nurses came for about three weeks, "so we could get some kind of familiarity with them." But, she added, "it's surprising. . . . Even with nurses that you think have done this a lot of times . . . I am more like the doctor telling them what to do. . . . And you know, even the doctors here . . ., you pretty much tell [them] . . . what you think needs to be done." According to this caregiver, "In a bigger city, they deal with it all the time," so although the interactions with home care nurses were "always good" and they were "very helpful," she always felt like "I'm the teacher, and they're learning from me."

Interestingly, some caregivers felt that they were expected to perform procedures beyond what medical professionals who later visited them were allowed to do. For example, I spoke with two different caregivers who had learned to change trachs, yet they told me that private duty nurses (licensed practical nurses, or LPNs) later assigned to them through Medicaid waivers were not trained to do so. One caregiver told me about suctioning her daughter's trach while riding in a medical ambulance because the emergency medical technicians (EMTs) were not trained in that procedure. These types of dynamics add stress for caregivers, who may not be able to fully rely on emergency medical services at home.

Caregivers Who Received Some Training in Hospitals

The training experiences of other caregivers in this book—those who did not have prolonged training in rehab facilities or hospitals—varied significantly. Some believed they learned a great deal before discharge, while others felt they did not. Of the caregivers who did receive training, some were actually allowed to perform procedures while still in the hospital.

Paul, for example, learned to attend to his wife's wound drains while the nurse watched and instructed him, giving him the opportunity to do the work himself. Beverly learned to give IV antibiotics in a large pediatric hospital. "They made me watch them for the first two, maybe three days," she recalled. "Then . . . they would slowly have me work into it. And of course, you know, you had to wash your hands real good first. And . . . they taught you how . . . when you open your alcohol things you never let it touch anything. I mean . . . they were very articulate . . . in their training. And . . . it was better for me to watch and observe and see how it was supposed to be done, than just be thrown into it and say, 'Here—you do it.' "

Although Beverly said the nurses in the hospital were patient with her for the most part, her training procedures were interrupted when personnel were in a hurry, as is clear from her description of a negative experience with one hospital nurse: "She really didn't want to give me the chance to do it. She wanted to do it, get it done, get out of there. . . . She wasn't patient and she just wanted to . . . be done with it, and move on to the next patient. But . . . the others, they were great." This example shows that even in an institution that has training procedures in place, individual actors may still affect the process. Although it is difficult to know for certain without interviewing the nurse involved, individual actions could be a response to institutional pressures to speed up work.

Some caregivers, particularly those who were in pediatric hospitals, were also allowed to practice on demonstration models ("dolls," "baby dolls," or "fake skin") before discharge. In these situations, hospital nurses generally supervised training and used a check-off sheet to indicate whether the procedures had been learned. Several nurses I interviewed emphasized that pediatric hospitals generally do a very good job of teaching because, as one nurse said, they realize the child may have an illness that lasts for an extended period of time. A home health nurse told me, "I've had children with trachs come home for the first time and they've just been taught so well. . . .—they know more than I do." Notably, although caregivers found this type of training to be helpful, they still had some anxiety about doing the procedures at home. As one mother commented, "Doing a procedure on a doll is not the same as doing it to your own kid."

Caregivers like Nancy were also allowed to practice with the types of pumps they would be receiving at home. "They did a pretty good job getting you ready," she said. "I mean they make sure you demonstrate your ability. . . . They make you go through the whole process. You know, setting up the IV, and getting the line ready." This experience contrasted greatly with that of caregivers who did not receive training on pumps in the hospital, and they explained that getting used to new equipment at home was very stressful.

Nancy, along with three other caregivers, also reported receiving written protocols, which gave detailed instructions on how to perform the procedures at home. According to Nancy, the protocol had "step by step what you needed to do . . . in case you're tired, you can't remember, your mind goes blank." These caregivers believed protocols helped a great deal with their execution of the labor.

Caregivers Who Received Little or No Training in Hospitals

Other caregivers' experiences varied significantly. Most reported that they did not receive written protocols on the procedures they were to perform at home. They were simply shown the procedures or talked through them by hospital nurses. For example, a husband who was learning to put formula in a feeding tube for his wife told me it was a "dry run" in the hospital—they pretended to pour the formula in the feeding tube.

Several of the caregivers who received little or no training in the hospital and were expected to perform intense care immediately upon discharge expressed feelings of being overwhelmed. Ava, who had to learn to irrigate her husband's wound, said the hospital nurse showed her the procedure only one time. According to Ava, the nurse drew up some saline in a syringe and shot it into a sink in the room but "really didn't invite me up there to see": "I thought, 'This can't be.' You know, because they're just showing me over a sink, a little sink, and I'm standing far *behind*. . . . She just called me over there and she said, 'You want to see how you do this? You just put this in here. Put . . . the water in it. Put this in here, press it and that's all you do.' I knew nothing after that. And I watched her and that was that. . . . I didn't know what she had done." In this case, Ava felt the nurse who showed her the irrigation procedure was not as caring as the other staff nurses. "Now if we would have had some of the other nurses that we had during that time," Ava told me, "they would have put me front and center and said, 'This is what you do. Grab it!'"

Again, hospital training processes appear to vary not only by institutional practices, but also by the particular nurses who are on a given shift and the amount of time they dedicate to teaching. As stated, this could be due to institutional pressures such as increased workloads and time constraints.

Notably, although caregivers who dealt with large pediatric hospitals were sometimes allowed to practice on models—if not the real person— this was not always the case. Meredith, for example, is a caregiver whose child requires total parenteral nutrition (TPN), a highly sterile technique that involves dispensing vital nutrition from a pump into a central line catheter. At the time of diagnosis, Meredith and her family lived in a large metropolitan area in the western United States. Although hospital personnel showed Meredith and her husband how to perform some procedures, such as changing the cap and dressing for their son's central line, they did not instruct them on how to operate the pump. "They want the nurses to handle everything," she said. Meredith described her feelings in the hospital and after discharge:

> When you're in the hospital, you're just watching and observing and learning all the lingo and what's happening, but you don't learn any of that [how to operate the pumps]. This is how we learned, and this kinda scares me. . . . The day he was discharged a nurse came to the house . . . and showed us how to spike the bag and "du da du" and all that, and run the pump and that was it. So we're . . . you know, there's no—there's paperwork on the pumps and how to run 'em and all—but—we're taking notes. I'm like, "Oh my God!" It's so scary, 'cause everything has to be so clean and sterile . . . and you're stressed out and [thinking], "What am I doing wrong?"

Morgan, who cared for her husband, also believed she did not receive proper instruction. She was required to learn several skilled procedures during the course of his illness, including the maintenance of a catheter and a feeding tube. She dealt with various providers, such as hospitals, nursing agencies, and equipment delivery companies, and felt that she was never given good instruction on how to perform the work:

> Well, what I heard several times in this process, or what I think I heard, was, well, you know, yeah, it's professional people that do this everywhere else, but since you're the caregiver, you've all of a sudden been knighted to be

able to do this—just because you have the title of caregiver. "Are you the primary caregiver?" "Yes." "Well then, you'll just do this." . . . I got that all the time. It's like, is that a degree? You know, I didn't go to school for this. So it . . . was just almost an unspoken—"It's somebody else's problem. It's not ours."

Caregivers who do not believe that they have received proper training undergo additional stress and may not feel qualified to perform the labor, at least initially. This may have repercussions throughout the skilled labor process. A home health nurse emphasized the importance of the hospital experience, which she described as having "the domino effect," saying, "If they had a bad experience in the hospital, then we get 'em—it just continues."

In terms of at-home learning experiences, caregivers also described processes that varied greatly in terms of the number of home health visits and the speed with which they were expected to learn. For example, Bridget was shown IVs once before discharge but wasn't allowed to practice. "They went through it with me one time and of course I still . . . didn't get it," she told me. Upon discharge, her husband was to receive four doses of medication a day—at 6:00 a.m., noon, 6:00 p.m., and midnight. When the home health nurse arrived, it was already time for the 6 p.m. dose, so the nurse did the procedure while explaining it to Bridget, thus leaving her to do the midnight and 6 a.m. doses on her own. Regarding the midnight dose, Bridget said she was "nervous! But I got it done. . . . I was so proud of myself. [*Laughs*.] You know, I could have sat down and cried!" Procedures done after normal business hours mean that nurses are often less available. This mismatch between bureaucratic work hours and the twenty-four-hour period in which work must be performed is a significant problem in the home health labor process (see also Ungerson 1990b). Moreover, caregivers indicated that although they knew nurses were on call, they felt tremendous pressure to perform procedures on their own. This topic will be addressed in greater detail in chapter 4.

Annette experienced a much more gradual learning process at home. She learned to change wet-to-dry dressings on a deep abdominal wound for her mother and was allowed to watch home health nurses perform the procedure several times before she actually did it herself. According to Annette, "I watched her—I don't know, maybe ten times. She would tell me what she was doing—as she was doing it, and afterwards I wrote stuff down." Annette said this process allowed her to compare her notes to the procedures being performed and ask questions. "If I forgot a step, I'd write it down, so that when I took over . . . I made sure I wasn't leaving anything out," she said. The fact that payer sources allowed these visits no doubt played a major part in her ability to learn over time. Annette said that at one point, the home health nurse was being "pushed" to release her mother, but that the nurse "fought" for the ability to keep coming out.

Importantly, some caregivers were sent home without having home health assigned, or they had trouble getting the instruction they needed to complete tasks. When Ava's husband was discharged without home health, she called her family doctor and he arranged it, but due to the delay, home health was not able to come for a few days. Fortunately, on their first day home, a family friend who was a nurse offered to help. She taught Ava how to irrigate the wound and Ava believed her to be a wonderful teacher. According to Ava, "She was just so gentle. . . . It was like with every word she said, she taught me something." The friend let Ava watch first before telling her to "take the point" of the syringe. Ava told me, "Even though I was holding it . . . she *guided* it and *that* helped me. *She* guided it so that I didn't have to put the point in there the first time. For some reason that helped me. . . . And I was doing it—but I wasn't at the same time—if that makes any sense." Ava said the difference between this type of instruction and that in the hospital was "just like night and day." Within a few days, home health arrived. Although Ava had a positive experience with them, and believed she learned much more about wound care and other procedures, she was very grateful that her friend was able to come immediately after hospital discharge. "Had she not been there that night, I would have been in trouble," Ava said.

Interestingly, two other caregivers said they learned how to do procedures from family members or friends who were nurses, and an additional three caregivers said they relied on nurse family members or friends for advice from time to time.[4] A few others said they benefited from having family members who worked in social services, who helped them understand what benefits they were entitled to. These cases illustrate how caregivers may be able to obtain resources and even additional instruction through personal ties. This linking of private and public worlds, however, is not possible for people without such connections.

The Question of "Willing and Able" Caregivers

As we have seen, caregivers come home with various experiences and knowledge levels. A number of issues stemming from structural factors, institutional arrangements, and communication patterns have the potential to impede the care work process. Based on their prior experiences working in multiple hospitals and institutions, many nurses believe that part of the reason that some families come home unprepared is that there is little time to teach in the hospital. Nurses "have so many things they have to get done in their eight hours," a nurse explained. Most acknowledged that hospital discharge planners—who are usually RNs or social workers—are in a tough position because they are often "stretched" in their responsibilities.[5]

Regardless of the training that families receive prior to discharge, nurses and administrators tell me that the goal of home health care is to make them "independent in their care"—meaning that nurses are to teach rather than provide care—and that one of the biggest requirements of the U.S. payer system is that there must be a "willing and able" caregiver in the home. Although hospitals are responsible for making sure that a willing and able caregiver is present, nurses indicated that they were sometimes skeptical that all care recipients really had such caregivers available. Nurses told me there are many situations in which they have to "try hard to find somebody," such as the case of a woman who needed multiple IVs and had no adult relatives in town, or a man who lived alone whose neighbor came four times a day to give him insulin injections and monitor his diabetes.

Although nurses related positive experiences in working with referring institutions, they also gave many examples of communication patterns between hospitals, families, and home health agencies presenting problems. Complicating the picture, sometimes information received from referral sources is very basic, perhaps just a list of medications or some demographic information. "If we could have more information, up front at least . . .—half an H and P [history and physical]—that would help," Josephine told me.

Nurses also acknowledged instances in which caregivers are under the false impression that home health nurses will actually come in and do all of the skilled care. "That's what they're told, but it's not [true]. . . . Medicare has been changing their guidelines and they don't want to pay the nurse to go every day," a nurse told me. A nurse administrator explained that caregivers in these situations are "put in a very tough spot. . . . They don't know really what they signed up for." This dynamic has caused some of the agencies to work more closely with discharge planners to ask for reassurance that families are informed about what they are expected to do.

Yet nurses also say that they believe the majority of caregivers they see *are* willing to learn because they believe that it is the best thing for the care recipient. "For the most part I think . . . family members, caregivers, are real receptive to learning," said Ruth, a home health nurse. Virtually all nurses say they look at the relationship between the caregiver and the care recipient as a key feature in their assessment of who will give good care. Vicky said, "I think people that . . . have a close relationship—they seem to want to *do* what they do. They want what's best for their family and most of them, if they have that sense, want to do it if they feel like that's what's needed." Indeed, as I will show in chapter 5, the caregivers in this book—all of whom performed skilled medical labor—spoke foremost about their relationship with their loved one in discussing the process of taking on skilled nursing, and many spoke out passionately against institutionalization. It was obvious that all saw care recipients as remarkably important people in their lives, and many expressed that they were glad they were able to help those they loved. Barbara said that she and her husband both prefer that he be at home when possible because of his important role in their children's lives: "We're kind of in our phase of life where as our children grow and they get older, we want to be at home. Mark wants to be at home, he doesn't want to be inpatient. If he can stay out of the hospital and get what he needs with home care, we're gonna do it."

The relationship dynamics and level of family support are key features of the skilled labor process, and will be explored more closely in chapter 4. Importantly, however, although self-assessment as to their readiness to do nursing work varied by caregiver (see for example the case of Paul in chapter 5), many stated that they were initially wary of performing procedures for which they did not have formal qualifications. A mother who had to give IVs to her child described her feelings when leaving the hospital: "It was pretty nerve-wracking 'cause you go home feeling that this is a nursing job . . . and I'm—I'm not a nurse. You know?"

Caregivers' assessment of their own skills was often quite emotional as they recounted—sometimes with wonder—the work that was necessary. A wife talked to me about her hesitation to go home from the hospital: "They were so sweet—those residents—I loved 'em. But I said, 'Are you sure he's well enough to go home?' And . . . of course I was hoping that he would say, 'Well maybe I'd better do a double take on this.'" Nurses, who acknowledge that the U.S. payer system places caregivers in hard situations, spoke frequently of their advocacy work in garnering additional resources or support, or locating family members, neighbors, or friends who were willing to help perform the procedures. They spoke of the critical need for family support. According to a nurse with a long career in home health,

> You can tell if the marriage is strained from the get-go . . . or you can tell if . . . the parents are fed up. . . . It could be that . . . you got an Alzheimer's [patient] and the caregiver is just damn worn out . . . and that is affecting whether they're able to do the care or are willing to do the care. And then you have to step in and help, you know? . . . How long has the caregiver been having to do this kind of stuff or *will* they have to be doing this kind of stuff? . . . They better have some support systems and if not, we need to sit down and talk about that.

Another nurse used the example of a daughter who feels "trapped" into having to do wound care, because she feels she "is the only one out there to do it." The nurse said that in such a situation, she monitors the case more closely and spans out her visits over time in order to assure patient safety. Moreover, although caregivers in this book said they enjoyed close relationships with care recipients, a few nurses said they have seen cases in which, due to the caregiver's body language or comments, they suspected women had felt trapped in relationships and did not feel like being attentive to their partner's needs. As one nurse said, "He lays there and she's okay with that, you know? . . . She's gonna do the limited amount." Nurses say that if they witness abusive or neglectful relationships, they have to draw in social agencies or protective services. According to a home health administrator, this is the most difficult situation they face. In speaking of cases involving elderly care recipients, she stated,

> If it's an abuse situation, we would have already had adult protective services involved, but we let them know we're having to discharge, and then

it's in their court. And *that* is the hardest situation we have. If it's an abuse
or neglect situation. . . . A lot of planning. A lot of thought . . . because . . .
no matter how bad it is in that home, [if] that client would rather stay there
than go to a nursing home . . . as long as they've been deemed *competent*,
and they are their own guardian, they can make that decision. . . . And we
have to walk away. Otherwise we're part of that neglectful situation. We're
enabling that situation more.

As is evidenced from these observations, serious issues surrounding the
structural and ideological components of placing labor on family caregivers cannot be denied. As Glazer (1993) observes, the U.S. health care
system sets up a workforce of paid and unpaid workers, and makes family
members into pseudonurses. Caregivers come into the medical labor process because of their relationship to care recipients, not because of their
proclivities toward this highly specialized work or their initial skills.

Moreover, there is a great deal of variance in skills training processes,
and the particular hospital experience impacts caregivers' orientation to
the labor, as well as their interactions with home health nurses. Once they
are home, although typical protocols such as observing a return demonstration appear common, there is much variability in teaching and learning styles, and payer sources play a prominent role in nurses' interactions,
as well as their ability to make teaching visits. The variation in these work
processes takes on even more meaning considering that caregivers have
multiple backgrounds and skill levels. It is the U.S. health system, and its
payer sources, that insists on "independence" and dictates the resources
to which caregivers are, or are not, entitled.

3

WHO PAYS?

My two careers have served me well in understanding how policy and social structure impact individuals' care work. As an accountant I understood the implications of market transactions within the U.S. economy. As a sociologist I understand how the social and health policies enacted by governments impact individual lives. Such insights are crucial in understanding the work of caregivers within the U.S. health care system.

My experiences as a caregiver have also given me a deep understanding of the importance of maintaining adequate health insurance, and the often emotional issues that arise as families face this challenge. Checking insurance deductibles, working with human resource departments and insurance carriers, opening bills that are shocking, and always carrying the fear of losing coverage are very real concerns. These play out differently for individuals based on many factors, such as their employment, their socioeconomic status, and their resources. Consideration of health benefits often structures major life decisions, such as where to live and where and how to work, and these decisions can cause great anxiety and insecurity.

There are good reasons for these concerns. U.S. health care is often criticized for being fragmented and inefficient. Scholars have demonstrated that the system has historically tied health benefits to employment, provided unequal access to care, incurred rising costs without associated health benefits, and placed a priority on for-profit players such as insurance companies, hospitals, and pharmaceutical companies (Eitzen, Zinn, and Smith 2014). Just after the time of my fieldwork, the 2010 Affordable Care Act (ACA) was passed. The ACA sought to increase the number of people with insurance and provide important consumer protections such as banning discrimination based on "preexisting" medical conditions, doing away with lifetime caps on coverage, and allowing children to remain on their parents' policies until age twenty-six (USDHHS 2018). These changes were desperately needed, yet at the time of this writing, the fate of the ACA was uncertain due to Republican efforts to "repeal and replace" it. (See the discussion below regarding recent changes and challenges to the ACA.)

While health care reform is a hotly debated topic, specific issues related to home health care have received far less attention. It is important to understand that payer sources structure home care labor in important ways. Medicare, state Medicaid laws, and private insurance policies determine the services that patients are entitled to and the number of visits that home health nurses can make. This greatly affects care work processes and the amount of unpaid labor that caregivers perform. Thus, in order to fully understand this impact, a fundamental knowledge of the major payer sources is essential.[1]

Medicare and Medicaid were both created in 1965 through Titles XVIII and XIX of the Social Security Act (CMS 2007) and are administered by the U.S. Department of Health and Human Services under the Centers for Medicare & Medicaid Services (CMS) (CMS 2007). There are significant differences between the two, however—not only in the funding source, but also in coverage and guidelines. Medicare is a federally funded program, while Medicaid is funded by both the federal and state governments, with expenditures making up a sizable portion of all state budgets. Unlike Medicare, Medicaid is managed by individual states based on federal guidelines that stipulate the services that must be provided to specific groups of poor individuals (CBO 2007, 18–19). As of the time of my fieldwork, the federal government required that "poor children and families who would have qualified for the former Aid to Families with Dependent Children program, certain other poor children and pregnant women, and elderly and disabled individuals who qualify for the Supplemental Security Income program" be covered (CBO 2007, 19). Many families and children who are on Medicaid are covered by Medicaid Managed Care plans, which have provider agreements with the state.[2] After my fieldwork, the Affordable Care Act provided federal funding for states to expand Medicaid eligibility for individuals whose income is 133 percent of the federal poverty level, although as of this writing, fourteen states had still not expanded coverage (Kaiser 2019).

Medicare has historically been a driving force in U.S. health policy due to its conversion of typical fee-for-service medical reimbursements into a standardized prospective payment system (PPS) (Mayes and Berenson 2006). In 1983, Congress's adoption of PPS meant that Medicare payments made to hospitals were based on standard predetermined groupings according to diagnosis—called diagnosis-related groups, or DRGs. This reimbursement system encouraged hospitals to discharge patients more quickly and transfer them to skilled nursing facilities, rehabilitation facilities, or home health agencies, which were still allowed to bill based on traditional reimbursement (Mayes and Berenson 2006, 99). This trend toward earlier hospital discharges, advances in medical technology, and allowance for "part-time or intermittent" care under Medicare guidelines resulted in dramatic growth in home health agencies in the late 1980s and early 1990s.[3]

This period of growth came to an abrupt halt, however, when Congress, in an effort to control costs, enacted the Balanced Budget Act of 1997. The act effectively changed reimbursements to home health agencies from a fee-for-service basis to an interim payment system (IPS) and finally to a PPS, which was fully implemented in 2000 (CMS 2010a). Medicare spending for home health fell from $14 billion to $9.2 billion between 1998 and 2000, due in part to the IPS, which contained a per-beneficiary limit (NAHC 2008, 3). Moreover, all services and supplies were bundled into one reimbursement, and blood draws were no longer eligible for home care services, unless performed in conjunction with another skilled medical procedure.[4] These changes resulted in significant downsizing and closing of home health agencies that had difficulty with implementation. The number of Medicare-certified home health agencies fell from 10,444 in 1997 to 6,861 in 2001 (NAHC 2008,10).

PPS, adopted in 2000, meant that now home health agencies, like hospitals, were paid fees prospectively based on home health resource groups, or HHRGs (similar to hospital DRGs). With the full implementation of PPS, the number of agencies grew steadily and reached 9,284 by 2007 (NAHC 2008, 10). The Balanced Budget Act and its mandated PPS brought significant changes to the industry, however. Rather than billing based on the number of visits to a home, successful agencies had to budget visits and supplies based on a prospective payment. This caused additional constraints in business practices. Several nurses who had been in practice before the PPS implementation lamented the change, remembering the times when they could make as many visits as they thought were necessary. One nurse said, "It was fee for service and you could provide whatever amount of care for however long." Another nurse administrator explained that under the old fee-for-service system, if she needed to go into a home "fifteen times" to teach, she could. But now, after PPS, "I have a diagnosis category and . . . the HHRG—which is the home health resource utilization group categories that determine how much I'm gonna get paid. So, for this same case, I may only get paid two thousand dollars but need to make fifteen visits . . . and you're paying the nurse sixty, seventy dollars a visit." As one home health nurse manager put it, rather than being paid for visits, "now a visit is an expense."

Medicare law also requires that in order to receive skilled services, a person must have at least one of the following medical needs: intermittent skilled nursing (other than just drawing blood), physical therapy, speech-language pathology services, or continued occupational therapy (CMS 2008, 36). Home health visits must be made by a Medicare-certified home health agency (CMS 2010b, 5). The person must also be "homebound," meaning that it is a "considerable and taxing effort" to leave home, although the guidelines do allow leaving for "medical treatment or short, infrequent absences," such as attending religious services (CMS 2008, 37).[5] Importantly, Medicare is designed for hospital stays and short-term rehabilitation stays—it does not cover long-term care.[6]

In contrast to Medicare, those on Medicaid generally have low income and few assets. States have flexibility to determine the exact eligibility rules, and there is great variability by state. During my fieldwork, nurses explained that patients who move across state borders may find that they are not eligible for the same benefits that they were before.

In order to better understand Medicaid eligibility for skilled home health nursing, I investigated the Medicaid rules in one midwestern state through discussions with Medicaid and home health administrators and caseworkers, a review of documents, and attendance at a state home health conference. In order to meet Medicaid requirements in that state, there had to be at least one skilled service per week, and the home health provider had to be a Medicare-certified home health agency. There were also specific time limits on combined skilled nursing and aide services. Services had to be "intermittent" and could not exceed more than eight hours per day and fourteen hours per week. The state, however, did allow for additional hours following a hospitalization, and had special considerations for children with a "comparable institutional level of care," regardless of whether they had had a hospital stay. Private duty nursing was also allowed if a person required continuous (rather than intermittent) skilled care and their needs met the state's guidelines.

Exploring state Medicaid rules reveals significant differences between Medicaid and Medicare guidelines. For example, although a person must be homebound in order to receive skilled nursing services under Medicare, this is not the case in the state-specific Medicaid laws I investigated. There were also differences in what nurses are allowed to do. In the state I analyzed, nurses are reimbursed for setting up pillboxes, but Medicare law did not allow this as a skilled service. Caregivers told me that under Medicaid, they are required to pick up their own supplies, but under Medicare, supplies are bundled and provided, although patients may have to pay out of pocket if they prefer a different type. Medicare also allows home health aides only for services that support skilled nursing care (CMS 2010b, 8–9), but states have various regulations and programs that may allow home health aides.

States can also apply for federal waivers that allow them to cover individuals who would ordinarily be excluded under Medicaid rules (CBO 2007, 3). In the midwestern state I investigated, a home health waiver was available for skilled nursing and other services for persons with severe medical conditions or disabilities—ones for which they may face institutionalization without such services. Thus, children with parents who have higher income than normally allowed under Medicaid could be granted a waiver if the child's medical need met state mandates. The number of slots for such waivers, however, is limited. As a hospital nurse with a long career in home health explained, "There are so many waiver slots per year . . . so it's unrealistic to think that if you have a new patient that's going home on a complex therapy that they would get a waiver. And we tell families that. We always tell them to apply for it, and . . . to see what happens, but there's no guarantee."

A review of private insurance further shows the complexity of allowable services for home health care. While Medicare and Medicaid have specific legal mandates for coverage, private insurance coverage is specified within the particular policy. Private insurers contract with employers or directly with consumers.[7] Insurance regulation has historically been left up to the states.[8]

Private health insurance varies widely in the United States, with some policies being much more generous than others. State variability in insurance can also be quite extreme,[9] and each state has their own standards as to which medical services health policies must cover. These "mandated benefits" vary widely and generally pertain to small group and individual markets (Kofman and Pollitz 2006,1–6; Bunce and Wieske 2009). As of 2009, twenty states had passed mandates for home health care and twelve states had passed mandates for hospice care (Bunce and Wieske 2009, 5). In an issue brief from the Commonwealth Fund, which conducts research on health issues, Frey and colleagues (2009) compared the state mandates for individual and small group policies with the Federal Employees Health Benefits Program (FEHBP) Blue Cross and Blue Shield standard benefits (similar to standard benefits offered by most large employer-sponsored plans) (Frey et al. 2009, 2). They concluded that in most cases FEHBP standards meet or exceed state mandates, but home health care is an exception. It has wide variability by state, with some states requiring greater coverage than what is in the FEHBP plan. For example, while the standard FEHBP covers home health nursing for two hours per day up to twenty-five days annually, home health mandates in Massachusetts require that insurers cover all home health services that are in accordance with a treatment plan, Wisconsin requires coverage for at least forty visits, and Texas covers sixty visits per year (4).

Notably, even after the 2010 passage of the ACA, with its ten essential health benefits (benefits that all policies must cover), there is still a great deal of flexibility by states in determining coverage according to state mandates. According to the National Conference of State Legislatures (NCSL

2018), this flexibility was increased when the CMS, under the Trump administration, issued a rule to "mitigate the harmful impacts of Obamacare [the ACA] and empower states to regulate their insurance market." What this actually involved was "a substantial change away from the benefit requirements in many health plans offered for 2014–2018" (NCSL 2018). Moreover, there is worry that the administration's defunding of subsidies, called cost sharing reductions (CSRs), may significantly impact those who buy insurance in the health care exchanges (NCSL 2018), and the Commonwealth Fund estimates that the 2017 repeal of the ACA's individual mandate—which requires that people purchase insurance—will result in "2.8 million to 13 million fewer Americans with coverage, and a 3% to 13% rise in premiums for bronze plans" (Eibner and Nowak 2018).[10] The administration's 2018 ruling increased insurance companies' ability to issue "short-term limited duration" policies, which do not have to comply with ACA essential benefits such as maternity care, or to offer protection for those with preexisting conditions (Pear 2018).[11] In the wake of these changes, advocacy to increase transparency and to assure adequate insurance for all has never been more important.

As we have seen, the differences in state regulations and mandates, as well as specific policy guidelines, mean that private insurance has significant variation. In regard to home health care, what we can say is that in general, home visits are limited and home health agencies must get approval for the number of visits they make. According to a nurse administrator, "They think something can be done in three visits. . . . 'That's all I'm gonna pay you, is three visits. You get it done and if you need more you have to call me and tell me.'"

These limitations have significant impacts on care recipients, and they structure the work processes for caregivers and nurses alike. In many cases, nurses told me about their advocacy work in speaking up to insurance companies on behalf of patients and caregivers. Calling for approval of extra visits if caregivers or patients needed more time to learn techniques or required additional support was a common theme—and this was sometimes a battle. Nurses said they must sometimes make the case that it is cheaper for home health to do the procedure than to pay for a readmission. As one put it, "'Do you want us to send them back to the hospital or nursing home? Then why don't you just give me the visit?'"

Though nurses said they were often able to arrange for more visits, and some said they had developed relationships with insurance providers that made the process smoother, this was not always the case. One nurse told me about being given one visit to teach an adult living alone how to do his own IV care, including changing the PICC line dressing. "I felt horrible," she said. ". . . That's a sterile procedure. . . . It was in the dominant hand and the insurance company authorized one visit."

It is also notable that in some cases Medicare and Medicaid coverage (depending on the particular state) may be more generous than health insurance policies. For example, discussions with administrators revealed that the type of private duty nursing services for those with continuous rather than intermittent needs, which are made available through Medicaid waivers, are generally not allowed by insurance companies, or are allowed for only short periods of time. It also appears that in some cases Medicare and Medicaid may allow more home health visits, and thus more time for teaching, than some insurance policies. Yet government health care in the United States is subject to legislative changes and may vary considerably as federal or state budgets experience cuts. Also, Medicaid covers those who live in poverty or are on waivers due to extreme medical disability, and this can pose additional issues of its own. For this book, nurses and home health administrators spoke about the slow-paying nature of Medicaid, particularly if it is managed by health maintenance organizations (HMOs). One caregiver said she had home care services dropped in her state because Medicaid did not reimburse the agency in a timely manner. The Medicaid reimbursement rate is also often lower than the rate for other payers, and according to social workers, those on Medicaid may experience more limits on providers and have difficulty crossing state borders to receive care. Medicaid is also tightly controlled. For example, caregivers said they needed prescriptions for every supply and that pharmacies would not fill medications until the caregivers had only a few days left. Said one, "They won't refill, depending on what the prescription is, until you have a minimum, like three days. So it's like, I'm in the pharmacy four out of five days a week." These examples demonstrate the complex and varying guidelines of U.S. payer sources and make clear the labor processes that are necessary to negotiate within their limitations.

Negotiating the System

Due to the system's complexity and the disparities in coverage among various payer sources, comparability of benefits in the United States is very difficult. In trying to decipher government benefits, one father said with an exasperated smile, "If you figure it out, let us know!" On several occasions, caregivers in this book referred to Medicare or Medicaid interchangeably, or didn't remember the specific names of the Medicaid waivers their loved ones were on. This is quite understandable. In the U.S. system, caregivers and patients are often unaware of the benefits they have or are entitled to.[12] Complicating this process is the historical cultural pervasiveness of individualist ideologies in the United States, which value personal responsibility and may result in caregivers feeling like they should be able to figure things out on their own.[13] The various guidelines also mean that reimbursement and billing processes are complex and require a great deal of documentation and coordination. In speaking about the often excessive amount of paperwork in home health care, one nurse confided to me, "It'll drown ya."

The fragmented nature of payer sources greatly affects patients and caregivers, who often negotiate systems with limited knowledge. While many of the caregivers I spoke with were glad to have "good" insurance, and the need to maintain such coverage was an important factor in making job-related decisions, there were difficulties when coverage was limited or denied. Some explained that insurance denials for preexisting conditions had been difficult for them or were potentially problematic if they wanted to move or change jobs. Hannah said that after her family moved for her husband's job, the insurance company accepted everyone except her son, who had a severe brain injury. "They accepted everybody except him— they said, due to the preexisting condition," she stated. "And . . . we had no medical care for him. And you know, he needed his seizure med and we couldn't afford it."[14] Another woman told me that her son, who had a spinal cord injury, was to be released from rehab even though he still had a bad bacterial infection. Their car ride home was three hours long, and she was afraid he would have an accident on the road and she would not be able to help him clean up in the car. She said it was a matter of being "observant enough to know . . . that is not gonna work . . . and standing up for yourself and saying, 'No we're not doing it.'" At her insistence, the insurance company ended up extending his stay for another week until the infection cleared.

Having multiple payer sources can also greatly complicate reimbursements, as in the case of a caregiver whose daughter was covered by her ex-husband's insurance policy as well as Medicaid. Medicaid would not approve an antibiotic to be administered at home until it got a decision by the insurance company first. The insurance company delayed its decision for three days, and the doctor finally said she would admit the child to the hospital if the company did not approve the antibiotic. After this standoff, the approval finally came. This mother said she felt as if she were "always fighting everything."

"Fighting" also came when applying for Medicaid waivers. Beverly had tried two to three times to get a waiver for her child but was turned down. She said, "I guess basically what it amounts to . . . is you're just put on a waiting list. Doesn't really matter what your need is, how critical your need is, how minimal your need is, you're just put on a waiting list and when a slot turns up . . . you know, it's just pick-a-number, stand-in-line kind of thing." Beverly did eventually receive a waiver after she applied tenaciously—filing an application one time per week, until her "number came up."

A large problem for people in this book, however, was that they didn't know about waivers and other services that were available to them and didn't apply for them when they could have. Isabelle was grateful that home health nurses told her about waivers and gave her advice on how to apply:

> They said, "No matter what, *do not* leave until you get with someone who has you fill out the application for the waiver." . . . They kept stressing that. . . . So I went down to the Medicaid office and then went through the whole process and . . . said, "I need to apply for the waiver." And they said, "We don't know what a waiver is." And I said, "Well they told me it's a Medicaid waiver for medically fragile children." They're just insisting, "No." And I said, "Can I talk to a supervisor?" And . . . so the supervisor came. She said, "Oh yeah, yeah, yeah, we do have waivers." So without the nursing agency telling me that . . . first of all I wouldn't have known to ask for it, and then if they would have said, "We don't have it" . . . I would have let it go. . . . Who knows how long it would have been before eventually I . . . found out?

Indeed, caregivers often found out about waivers in serendipitous ways—from acquaintances, family members, or others. Adrienne cared for her adult son, who had a severe brain injury, for four and a half years before finding out from a social worker at a doctor's visit that he was eligible for a waiver. In addition, if she agreed to take classes and train as a nurse's aide, she could be paid for some of her care work through a state program. She said she "had no clue" these services were available and would have appreciated knowing because her son, since his accident, had experienced extreme financial difficulties leading to bankruptcy.[15]

The worry over insurance coverage was also a major concern for care recipients who were struggling to maintain productive lives. Some expressed disappointment that insurance would often limit service provision or even refuse to pay, which made it difficult for them to maintain their independence. Grant, who sustained a spinal cord injury and was able to work, paid for Medicaid insurance in his state but was upset that his insurance would no longer cover his rehab. While they would pay to "take care of a problem," they would not pay for preventative services—"They don't want to help you not get to that problem," he said. He had also tried to work with his local YMCA to get more equipment for people in wheelchairs, but "they always say they can't afford it," he told me. Tessa was concerned because she was recently discontinued for disability Medicaid, which was her secondary insurance: "I had no idea why they cut me off. . . . I mean I have a disability but they have other requirements besides the fact I'm in a wheelchair. . . . The reason why they said that I don't qualify is 'cause I can potentially carry a full-time job."

Issues related to balancing health insurance and attempting to work are very difficult for care recipients. Even attempting to work part time was challenging to Mark, a father who eventually went on disability. Although Mark said that he really wanted to "contribute to society," he felt that this was difficult because the welfare system was either "all or nothing." Thus, while working to maintain independence, care recipients often must negotiate systems that force them to consider the money and benefits they could earn in the labor market, their insurance requirements, and the need to take care of their health. This can be a challenging navigation.

It is clear that having ample insurance available for all people, without stratification by the payer source, is essential. The protections under the ACA, which prohibit discrimination based on so-called preexisting conditions, must be upheld, and the historical practice of tying health insurance to jobs is clearly a no-win situation. When people are experiencing an illness they often are unable to work, and caregivers may be precluded from full-time work as well.

Currently, the multiple-payer system promotes confusion, additional stress, and uncertainty. Health policy should focus on systems that are effective and comprehensive, and that promote an understanding of benefits. Medicare, for example, while not without shortcomings, is a national system that has benefited Americans greatly due to its transportability across state borders and its standard benefits. This allows caregivers and care recipients in multiple states to better understand their benefits, to plan, and to advocate for specific coverage. National comprehensive coverage that streamlines payment processes, has transparency, and allows for comparability is a crucial need for all Americans.

Part II

Relationships, Identities, and Emotions in Skilled Family Care Work

4

Integrating Care Work with Life

I was in my son's bedroom. We had just moved. Boxes were everywhere. My parents had driven up to help after my son's second hospital admission. We listened carefully to the nurse's instruction. My mother and I took notes. The nurse left. I was administering the first IV on our own, with my parents hunched over me. It was near dark outside. As I prepared the IV my dad warned, "Watch the bubbles—I heard they can go up to the brain." I looked daggers at him, but after that, I never neglected to watch for those bubbles.

In my experience, carrying out skilled medical procedures at home was challenging. We juggled schedules, set alarm clocks, organized supplies, and—amid regular household chores and activities—prioritized the careful injection of IV antibiotics over everything else. My discussions with caregivers reified the often dynamic nature of integrating skilled care delivery into home life. While some tended to care recipients with mobility issues and spent limited time outside the home, others administered skilled care in various places, including parking lots, schools, and church pews.

I have often wondered how many backpacks, or coolers in the trunks of cars, contain life-saving medicines and supplies—ready for injection, ingestion, or inhalation. Skilled care, it seems, is happening all around us. And caregivers may have various feelings of competency and preparedness; some may be balancing on an emotional tightrope.

Although there is scant literature regarding the labor processes in at-home skilled care work, we do know that home health, in general, involves a renegotiation of existing space, new rituals, and a certain amount of trial and error (Albert 1990; Corbin and Strauss 1990; Twigg 1999). Homes, by their nature, vary greatly, and the performance of nursing work often brings in multiple actors, such as nurses, therapists, and aides, which can create new negotiations for caregivers and also result in a loss of privacy (Murphy 1991; Twigg 1999). In order to accommodate medical interventions, homes may require modification and equipment (Corbin and Strauss 1988, 92–93), and this can often violate notions of order and cleanliness (Angus et al. 2005). In a study in Quebec, Canada, researchers found that transfers of "high-tech" medical care to homes were "trivialized" and made without a careful consideration of the context and condition of the home, the need to prepare for the unexpected, and the importance of patients and families having adequate knowledge and sufficiently integrating information about the condition or disease (Guberman et al. 2005).[1] Moreover, Guberman and colleagues point out that discharge policies do not always consider the home's physical, psychological, and social environment, and the anxiety caused by performing procedures without supervision or backup (Guberman et al. 2005).

There are significant differences between the work structure of unpaid family caregivers and that of medical professionals who work in a hospital or other institution. Unlike professionals, family caregivers do not have workplace protections, such as colleagues to cover while they are ill, professional networks, or the possibility for worker organization (Ungerson 1990b, 24). They are not protected by labor laws such as the Fair Labor Standards Act, which sets a federal minimum wage, or other important legislation that provides resources for paid workers (Duffy, Armenia, and Stacey 2015, 12). The division of labor is also vastly different. At home, one or a few people carry out caregiving work, whereas professionals in bureaucratic settings have a larger division of labor and set work hours (Ungerson 1990b, 24). Although some family caregivers can receive compensation under state Medicaid waiver programs (see Stacey and Ayers 2012, 50–51; and chapter 3 of this volume), they work without professional status, and in the United States they have systematically been excluded from compensation and denied state subsidies.[2] Work performed at home has been so devalued that even paid home care workers—those who perform body care and tending—have been repeatedly left out of labor law protections (Glenn 2010, 129; Boris and Klein 2012, 4–18). Their struggle to maintain a living wage has often been at odds with the cultural fear that care recipients would be unable to afford care (Boris and Klein 2012, 8).

Because family caregivers work at home and are often unpaid, much less is known about the work they do. By interviewing caregivers, I hoped to see how they dealt with implementing skilled nursing labor in their home lives. I wanted to better understand the practical and interactional components of the labor. How did caregivers organize themselves to get the procedures done in a timely and accurate matter? Did they feel competent in the work they performed? What obstacles did they face? I also wanted to know how the work interfaced with existing family relationships and the resources that were available in homes.

Home as a Place of Care Work

Homes, by their very nature, lack the resources and support of a hospital, and often geography—the physical separation between the home and the hospital—places obstacles in the coordination of care. Several caregivers told me of frenzied trips to ERs, sometimes an hour or more away, when equipment malfunctioned. Moreover, although caregivers reported many positive interactions with home health nurses, frustration and scheduling difficulties with home health agencies were not uncommon. One caregiver told me she met resistance in trying to schedule agency visits: "When I would call, they would always say, 'Well you live so far away.'" Another caregiver reported "no shows" and had to fire the agency. He stated, "They told you when they were going to be there. What you needed had absolutely nothing to do with it."

Unlike bureaucratic settings, which have standard work shifts, care work at home takes place over a twenty-four-hour period (Ungerson 1990b, 24), and caregivers' schedules are completely different from the schedules of the organizations they depend on for resources, such as delivery companies, vendors, or pharmacies.[3] A home health nurse I interviewed observed this mismatch when she told me about her frustration when patients are discharged "at ten o'clock at night from the hospital for IV therapy" with only a prescription. Noting the late hour, she said, "A prescription, what am I supposed to do with that?" Many of the nursing agencies themselves also prioritize workday hours, with on-call nurses coming out "after hours" only if absolutely necessary.

As is evident from contrasting the bustle of a busy hospital with the atmosphere in many homes, the division of labor and the people who do it are entirely different. In the hospital, nurses work in shifts to provide patient care. At home, there are far fewer people available, and they are in deeply embedded, preestablished familial roles and relationships, as well as existing patterns of housework and childcare. A nurse who has extensive experience working with families and children talked about how much work mothers perform at home, and how this should be factored into the amount of caregiving they can reasonably be expected to do: "I think that's another thing that people at the institution don't even think about. . . . You know, 'If you can do home care—go do home care.' I said, 'Wait a minute, she's already doing this, this, this, and this. . . . You think she can add one more thing on? When she's supposed to sleep? . . . I want you to go home with this mom and try to do everything she does for twenty-four hours.' It's like, 'I can't do that.' I'm like, 'No kidding, so that's why *she* can't do it, you know?'"

Because home is oriented toward relationships, "private" activities, and provisioning (DeVault 1991), rather than toward bureaucratic standards, compliance with medical regimens can also be more difficult. Several caregivers I interviewed worried when care recipients didn't take medicine as they should, didn't eat enough to regain strength, or didn't do therapies when they were supposed to. Caregivers said they had to walk a fine line because they did not want to nag and pressure; yet they also did not want the care recipient to become ill. According to a father, "You gotta observe . . . and watch and let them have enough rope to either . . . do it right or hang." Caregivers' emotional attachment to care recipients can also complicate compliance. Adrienne said she felt guilty when she made her son, who has a brain injury, do therapies that she knew hurt him. "Your heart breaks; you feel guilty 'cause you're making him do it."

Another primary way that medical labor impacts family life is that hospital-sized equipment is now located in a family's living space—space that was not originally designed to accommodate a plethora of pumps, hospital beds, or other devices.[4] Organizing supplies and managing logistics can be challenging. As a mother said to me, "Where am I gonna put this stuff? . . . How am I gonna keep it clean? . . . How am I gonna keep my [other child] . . . out of it?" Keeping home and hospital separate was an ongoing challenge. Barbara explained, "We try to keep everything put away or in one spot . . . so it's not all over the place. And we have certain spots that we keep certain things and that helps." Yet while some caregivers negotiated tension by the delineation of the medical and nonmedical (Angus et al. 2005, 168–74), others eventually relaxed such boundaries.[5] As she showed me her garage refrigerator, Meredith poked fun at her family's initial resolve that it was to be used only for her son's medical supplies. Her husband had originally declared, "Nothing else can go in here!" But now, she joked, "the beer's in there too."

Sometimes, though, bringing home medical supplies caused real dilemmas when the home did not have enough space to accommodate them, as Alice explained:

> I lived in a little two-bedroom apartment. And to get in . . . you had to go up on one step, which was very difficult with a wheelchair. . . . My neighbors helped me around as far as getting [my daughter] in and out, holding the door for me, and that type of thing. But . . . it was tough . . . because her hospital bed was in my living room. . . . All of her supplies were in my living room. . . . There was no room for anything. And if she was in her wheelchair, you couldn't get around. . . . There was just no way. No room whatsoever.

Alice's family later moved in order to have more room and better accommodate medical equipment. Indeed, caregivers from five other families told me they had moved either to find more adequate space, to move in with adult care recipients, or to be closer to quality care. Caregivers from seven additional families reported significant changes to their homes, including widened doors, ramps, or changes to the floor plan. I toured some of them and saw how clever families were at integrating Hoyer lifts, vents, and suction machines with sofas, dining tables, and other furniture.

Another issue was that—unlike in a hospital, where supplies and equipment are readily available—at home supplies must be ordered and delivered. A nurse I interviewed shared the challenges of coordinating supplies and services in home care. "Nothing is fast at home," she told me. Some caregivers reported unacceptable delays in delivery or said they had received equipment that didn't work. Supplies may also come from multiple sources, which can complicate delivery. A mother told me that when parts came from different areas of the United States, it got "really confusing." She said, "The people who are taking these orders do not know anything about supplies. . . . We keep getting the wrong supplies and they won't take it back."

Supplies may also come in different packages or have different designs than caregivers are used to. A husband caring for his wife shared his frustration in trying to replace a feeding tube piece when the "three-way snap-shut gizmo that you put . . . the syringe tube into . . . got nasty" and needed to be replaced. "Nobody could find the same piece," he said. Caregivers also experienced difficulties when payer sources, bureaucracies, or institutions determined the types or number of supplies that were allowed. (See chapter 3 for a discussion of payer sources.) Medicaid would not allow one woman to refill prescriptions until she had a minimum number on hand and would not work with her so she could condense trips to the pharmacy. A mother expressed her frustration about a recent change to a new home health company:

> When we changed home care companies, we get brand new pumps we don't know how to use. So someone's gotta come out, teach us how to use the pumps . . . go over the manual. Different tubes . . . they stop carrying this certain manufacturer tubing so we get a brand new [one]. . . . And I hate the one we have now 'cause . . . for some reason . . . it kinks, so that's why he was beeping off every two hours last night. And . . . home care companies carry different products. I hate the caps that our home care company uses now. Hate them.

Some caregivers also had issues when supplies were delivered that they didn't know how to use. Discussing a suction machine, a caregiver told me, "It was delivered to my house . . . by whoever delivers suction machines. A lot of times, what they do, these companies . . . will send out the machine and the person that delivers it is a delivery person. They have no idea. They can set it up, but they don't instruct you." Some caregivers said they ended up reading the manuals or trying to figure out the machines with other family members, which Hannah described as "muddling through" to "try to see what works."

The physical environment of the home itself also posed challenges, and many caregivers expressed great worry about keeping the house free of germs. Several described strict processes such as "scrubbing down" entire areas, and one caregiver said that her family was so worried about cleanliness that they made a family member who was a plumber strip at the door. In caring for those with breathing issues, some caregivers took extra precautions, such as keeping live plants out of the house, or changing showerheads more often to reduce bacteria. These protocols became part of home life.

A few caregivers realized they may have been excessively worried about cleanliness, which is understandable in light of incomplete information. Annette, for example, said she and her family "went too far" because they didn't know how much was enough: "We kept the house sterilized. We wiped down everything. . . . Her first time through chemo . . . we would sterilize the bathroom. . . . When she was done, we'd get her out of the bathroom, take her back to bed, hold our breath, flush the toilet, and run out. We couldn't shut the lid because she had a great big toilet seat on there. . . . And that was crazy, we didn't need to go that far, but nobody told us that we didn't need to do that. We didn't ask that."

The caregivers' accounts of cleanliness are important because they reveal how personal understandings can greatly impact the care process. Indeed, the nurses I interviewed said that educating families about germs and the importance of maintaining clean supplies is an important part of their job. Although they believe that in most cases care recipients are better off at home, where they are not exposed to hospital antibiotic-resistant bacteria, they also noted that homes do vary significantly in terms of organization and cleanliness. While they said they do not make value judgments about this, and that their primary concern is safety, they do sometimes witness situations where supplies are not organized or protected and it is necessary to confront the family. In a home, a nurse told me, there are "so many things we can't control. . . . It could be absolutely a horribly filthy situation." Nurses also said they may have to improvise depending on the resources available—by boiling water on the stove if there is no hot water, using hand sanitizer if there is no running water, or taking extra precautions if there is a problem such as insect infestation— for instance, not sitting on furniture, changing smocks between houses, or not taking their bags into the house.[6] The possible effects of varying home environments in the skilled labor process is an important dimension of care work—and one that deserves further study, especially given the magnitude of skills that are performed at home.

The fact that caregivers performed "skills" that were not legally allowed to be carried out by agency aides and other workers also caused coordination issues for some caregivers. A caregiver who experienced health problems himself ended up hiring people who were not nurses to help him because agency aides were not allowed to perform skilled procedures, such as administering a feeding tube. "The thing that I would really consider the most complicated . . . comes down more to a legal issue," he said. "We had all kinds of different caregivers that I was trying to hire from agencies and we ended up with our own—private—we just hired predictable people—because you couldn't get people from an agency to *do* anything. They were either gonna send you an aide who wasn't allowed to touch squat . . . or a nurse who wasn't gonna *stay* there, so . . . really it was . . . frustrating."

Although this caregiver was able to pay out of pocket for additional help, his dilemma shows how skilled caregivers' needs may fall through traditional legal cracks. Aides also face dilemmas in these situations because they feel pressured to respond to skilled needs, but they are not legally allowed to do so (see Stone 2001; Stacey 2005, 841–42).

Flying Solo: Feelings of Competency and Self-Evaluation in the Home

Whether or not caregivers received training in the hospital or rehab, most said they were still very anxious, sometimes even overwhelmed and frightened, the first time they had to perform procedures by themselves at home. Elle explained, "You got *all* these supplies sitting out there and you're thinking to yourself, 'I will *never*, you know, I'm gonna kill my kid. I am *never* gonna be able to do this, not break sterile technique. . . . I'm gonna get these drugs confused . . . air's gonna end up in the line.' You know, a million things."

Indeed, some caregivers did describe making mistakes. A wife who was giving IVs to her husband "felt like a dirty dog" when she overslept, and a mother "freaked out" when she realized she had administered lipids at too fast a rate, which she knew could potentially harm her son's liver. Both caregivers said they immediately contacted home health, who talked them through the situation and assured them that the care recipient would be okay.

Caregivers dealt not only with the medical procedures, however, but also with their feelings about the care recipient's overall health and prognosis, and whether the recipient would be able to adapt to new regimens. The emotionality of these processes cannot be overstated. (See chapter 5 for a discussion of emotion work.) Besides providing professional-level medical labor, caregivers also had to perform what Folbre and Wright (2012, 4–5) refer to as "support care"—making sure the house was clean and organized, providing food and supplies, and filling prescriptions. The multiplicity of tasks was overwhelming to some of the caregivers. A caregiver who was given only minimal instruction before discharge and was not assigned home health care had a friend come to stay with her husband so she could go out and get supplies. She said she "sobbed" and "screamed all the way to . . . the pharmacy to get the prescriptions, and to get the food."

Despite their initial anxiety, however, many caregivers said they were glad to be home, because they did not want their loved ones to be in hospitals or institutions.[7] Over time they developed strategies to get their arms around the routine. Some, like Rita, wrote down lists of medications, or made to-do lists. Others made charts or kept detailed medical records in computer files. Several said that the work itself required a great deal of concentration and that it was necessary to "really focus." It was, according to Faye, "like clockwork": "As long as you get into a routine, then it's not as overwhelming," she said. She, like many other caregivers, told me, "You just take one step at a time." Phoebe, a single mom who cares for her child who had a spinal cord injury, said she takes things "one day at a time . . . sometimes one minute at a time." Virtually all caregivers, even those who were tentative or who second-guessed their own competency, believed their ability to do the job increased over time. Some said that new procedures became easier to learn once initial skills were mastered, while others, who performed multiple procedures, questioned their effectiveness in certain procedures but not others.

A common theme was the importance of planning. Several caregivers spoke of gathering supplies ahead of time and allowing themselves enough time to "do it right." As Paul put it, "There's only one thing you can do at a time successfully and so you have to allocate a time slot."

The best place to perform procedures depended on equipment and timing; for example, IV antibiotics or tube feedings done at night were most often performed in the care recipient's bedroom. Skilled medical care involved intense monitoring that called for a great deal of judgment and troubleshooting. Paul said he relied on a range of health indicators to see whether he needed to call a medical professional for help. "I knew what the ranges were," he told me. "Blood pressure, temperature. . . . Is her pulse racing?" Some caregivers worried because it was difficult to tell whether problems were truly significant, especially if a care recipient had cognitive or physical issues that interfered with his or her ability to express pain. Hannah felt guilty that it took almost six months for doctors to diagnose her son's gallbladder problem because he was unable to tell them specifically about his pain. "Leading up to [the diagnosis] was very, very frustrating and difficult," she said.

Sleep patterns were also disrupted. One mother described the routine when she gave IVs:

> I feel strongly that if you're gonna heal and get better, you need to sleep. . . . So my window of opportunity to sleep, really for eighteen months, was from like midnight to . . . well I had to get the drug—the drug had to be . . . out of the refrigerator and at room temperature before we started the infusion. So . . . I could get to bed at twelve-fifteen and get up at four to get the [drug] out of the refrigerator . . . then get back up at five to start that infusion.

Clearly this meant that caregivers prioritized their loved one's sleep over their own. Elle said that she "charged up for those periods of time" when procedures were needed, and Nancy said, "I have my breakdown afterwards."

Some caregivers turned their loved ones as much as every two hours to prevent bedsores, others said they stayed awake to make sure they could still hear their loved ones breathing, and still others changed sleeping arrangements in order to be close by. According to Bill, "It was a matter of claiming out space at the foot of my bed for [my nephew's] hospital bed." Bridget said her husband began sleeping downstairs on a chair. "He never slept on the bed, he couldn't," she told me. When she became afraid that she couldn't hear him, she said, "I got to where . . . I slept downstairs on the couch." Caregivers reported using wireless doorbells, baby monitors, or cell phones so loved ones could call for help if they needed it.

The extent of caregivers' evaluation by medical professionals varied once they arrived home. Paul, who took care of his wife's wound and drains, said he received additional evaluations from home health nurses after her subsequent surgeries. He told me, "They twice came in during that four-month period and watched me do everything and said, 'You're doing what we could do. . . . It looks okay to us.'" When I asked Paul if he felt like he was doing a good job he said, "Absolutely. . . . If there was any doubt in my mind I would have called. . . . I would not have let that go by the boards." For Isabelle and Randy, who worked with home health nurses over time to learn their son's trach and feeding tube care, the nursing agency felt they were doing such a good job that the agency asked them if they would be willing to mentor some of the LPN waiver nurses—a fact that speaks volumes about the unpaid labor these caregivers provide.

Some of the caregivers, however, felt they received very little feedback once they were home. If they did receive some type of evaluation, it was only because they knew that home health nurses were documenting their competency in the chart. As one caregiver said, the evaluation "was never direct." Individual variances in feelings of competency are paramount in considering the skilled care process. For some, doing the procedure once or a few times in the presence of a nurse seemed to be enough, while others felt they needed more time to learn—particularly if they believed their work was very complex. For Morgan, who had to perform multiple skilled procedures in caring for her husband, a nurse observing her doing a procedure once was not enough. "I never did it the first time," she said. "I mean people say, 'Oh you did really well,' and they think, 'I'm done.' Well gosh, let's take that off and try it again—see if I can do it well two times. They don't give you that opportunity."

Like me, the caregivers in this book said they felt a tremendous amount of responsibility to perform procedures correctly, and many described intense self-evaluation processes. According to Simon, who along with his wife cared for their son, coming home from rehab was a period of "no rest": "It was always . . . a constant worry. 'Are we doing everything?' . . . There was always something going wrong; we made two or three steps forward and then five steps backward." Doing what Phoebe called "the stuff" meant, she said, asking the question, "Did I do it right? Did I . . . do everything that I was supposed to do?" Some caregivers looked to assessments from care recipients themselves to know whether things seemed to be going right. A caregiver said she felt confident when her husband told her, "From now on, I don't want anyone doing the trach except for you. . . . *You* get the seal right."

Importantly, caregivers often looked to medical outcomes or doctors' assessments of the care recipient's condition as a test of their abilities. In instances where outcomes were measurable, caregivers knew that what they were doing seemed to be working. When I asked Annette if she felt like she was doing a good job in the wound care she performed, she said that they could "see a difference." When home health nurses came to the house, "they always measured it, so you could tell." According to Gail, a mother who takes care of her son following his spinal cord injury, "We've had like what—two doctors—tell us that we . . . take really good care of him. . . . I guess that makes you feel good, you know? We must have been doing something right."

This judgment of performance based on medical assessments, however, can place additional worry on caregivers, who are often dealing with very serious conditions that despite all their efforts are difficult to manage. Although she tried to do everything very carefully for her son's in-and-out catheter, a mother explained that she could not prevent his infections, so they eventually had an indwelling catheter placed. "No matter how sterile I made it," she said, "no matter how . . . careful I was . . .—he kept getting infections. So we had to go to the doctor and take care of it."

In some cases, caregivers' own health problems made it more difficult to administer care. Sidney felt bad because he believed his back injuries interfered with his ability to provide care for his wife. "Twice I had to call my neighbors because . . . she slipped and I couldn't get her back up by myself. . . . It was very frustrating when I could physically *not* do certain things." Indeed, five caregivers reported injuries or illnesses that made it more difficult to perform the care work.

Moreover, although virtually all caregivers said they knew they could call home health nurses for advice when they needed it, they also told of times when talking over the phone went only so far. When a mother accidentally pushed air into her child's IV, she said she tried really hard "to stay very calm" as she dialed the home health agency. The nurse who answered told her to pull back on the IV line and get the air out—and then the nurse hung up. Shocked at the amount of force necessary to pull back, the caregiver was afraid she would "turn his arm inside out," and she was also alarmed because the blood looked "real choppy." She called the home health agency three times to work through the problem, and although the PICC line was checked the next day in a doctor's clinic and found to be in good working order, she was nonetheless deeply affected by the experience. In the hospital, patients have the benefit of the knowledge and skill of not only one professional but many. Registered nurses or other health care professionals and staff can compare one case to others. If there are questions, there are other people—not just colleagues but also supervisors—to consult. This kind of expertise is not available in the home.

Relationships, Home Work, and Home Economics

Caregivers shared many experiences that attest to the dynamic nature of the home. Some care for young children, who, in addition to complying with strict medical regimens, have to do routine childhood activities such as attending school and participating in events. According to Nancy, even though there is a lot to do in terms of taking care of her daughter's health, "She's still a kid, and she's gotta take a bath and she's gotta do homework and she's gotta get all that other stuff done."

Caregivers also talked about the importance of preparing and organizing meals (which was sometimes more challenging due to special diets or the need to puree food), maintaining activities with other children, and trying to attend social functions or fulfill personal commitments. While it is true that many caregivers said they curtailed their own social activities, especially in cases where care recipients were not mobile, the presence of other children often greatly increased activity. According to Barbara, who helps care for her husband as well as her two children, "You're going about your everyday life trying to keep it all together."

The experience of care work can vary greatly depending on such factors as the amount of housework or skilled care taken on by partners or spouses, other family members who provide backup help, the duration of care, and the age, health, and independence of the care recipient. Some caregivers were able to maintain full-time jobs and take off only during periods of illness, while others—due to factors such as the severity of the condition, employer inflexibility, or multiple caregiving roles—were not. Not surprisingly, caregivers who had good jobs, had flexible work schedules or understanding bosses, were able to work from home or the hospital, or were able to take leave under the Family and Medical Leave Act (FMLA) or other leave, were better off. Four families were able to pay out of pocket to hire caregivers or other helpers on a part-time basis.

Five caregivers took care of care recipients at the end of life. These were intense and emotional but also time-limited periods. Others took care of those with cognitive or physical problems, which required ongoing assistance. Caregivers who were in this situation worried about the future of the care recipient's health, particularly in cases of cognitive impairments, when they may not be able to speak up effectively for themselves. Adrienne takes care of her adult son who has a severe brain injury, and worries, "Who's gonna take care of him when I'm gone?"

Other care recipients were able to eventually achieve independence with some or all of the procedures, or no longer needed certain procedures. Marcus lives at home with his parents and told me he is mostly independent in his care. "I can pretty much take care of myself. . . . If I can do it, I'm gonna do it," he said.

Some care recipients learned to take care of their own catheters or colostomies, to administer some of their own IVs, or to help organize and direct their care. A ten-year-old was able to take over her insulin management under supervision, and a teenager learned how to place an NG-tube over time. Although a mother primes the pump for her teenage son's feeding tube, he actually hooks himself up to the tubing. She said, "He doesn't let me touch that, which is fine, because you know I can't feel that. . . . It'd be like somebody else changing my earring."

As seen in the introduction to this book, we know that there are important patterns in caregiving labor, and it is women who are most often caregivers. Gender influences preexisting family dynamics, relationship patterns, and divisions of labor within the family, and there are also strong societal expectations that women are the "natural" ones to assume such care (Cancian and Oliker 2000; Daniels 1987). Prior scholarship has also shown that care work may not only affect caregivers' ability to work outside the home; it may reorder other household work, such as laundry, cleaning, and childcare.[8] Although men's participation in housework is increasing, when women are in the home, they usually perform most of this kind of work.[9] This pattern holds even when women are employed outside the home, resulting in a "second shift" of women's labor (Hochschild with Machung 1989). Moreover, women often downplay their work at home (DeVault 1991).

Generally, the women in this book performed more of the skilled medical care for children within their families as well as the day-to-day care, such as getting children to medical appointments and ensuring compliance with medical regimens. As in other studies of household labor (see Coltrane 2000), the women also took greater responsibility for organizing the labor, even when their husbands helped a great deal—for example, women caregivers of children were likely to make lists or tell their husbands the specific things that needed to be done.[10] In general, it was women who took the lead in learning and performing procedures even if they worked outside the home. Although some of the men took off work using vacation days, FMLA, or paternity leave, women took off more time from work and were more likely to work part time or stay out of the workforce for longer periods.

Social support varied by each household.[11] Some families had good support systems, especially for "support care" (Folbre and Wright 2012, 4–5). Several said that family, friends, neighbors, and church members visited, brought food, babysat, mowed grass, helped build ramps, arrived to listen to home health nurse instruction, provided emotional support, or helped with fundraising activities. Other caregivers had limited social support. Nurses said that in their experience, this variation is not uncommon. As one told me, "You see good family support and then you see some people that have *no* family support." Nurses also reported cases where care recipients are home alone, either because the caregiver doesn't live there or because there is no caregiver available. Some of these care recipients may live in challenging situations. One nurse said, "We've gotten to a house before and maybe somebody lives by themselves, doesn't have anybody dependable to come . . . or that would be compliant with coming every time . . . and the home environment isn't as clean as it should be for getting therapy. . . . You can be surprised to look at someone . . . and their home environment might look so much worse than you might think."

Nurses say that these cases involve, as one put it, "calling the insurance companies" and telling them, and the cases demonstrate the variability in family situations and the dangers of assuming that all patients have caregivers ready and available.

Although gender norms were apparent in my study, there were several cases of couples in which partners or husbands shared a great deal of the skilled work for their children. Three of the men interviewed who helped their spouses care for children took turns performing procedures and rotated nights in monitoring pumps at home or for hospital stays. Two men were the primary caregivers for their ill spouses, and their stories give rich insight into the performance of such labor. In both cases these men lived alone with their spouses and had no adult children nearby. Although one did have other family members close, he saw caregiving as his responsibility. As would be expected, in cases of partners who are in relationships with strong norms of reciprocity, performing the work appears to be a way of demonstrating commitment and dignity.

The particular family formation plays a prominent role in who is available to do the work. Caregivers who are caring for spouses face difficulties because they must shoulder a great deal of the skilled labor, may also need to work outside the home, and may not have immediate family members available to help (Oliver 1983; Corbin and Strauss 1988, 112–13). This can be especially hard if the caregiver is economically vulnerable, as in the case of a wife who used FMLA to care for her husband, but was then fired because her employer would not allow her to work part time. In some households, as we have seen, care recipients may even live alone. It may be that they value independence, but not having others nearby can greatly complicate the care process. Moreover, although some caregivers expressed that they did not want to make the siblings or children of care recipients responsible for care, sometimes in cases of single parents or small families with children, teenagers or siblings—both boys and girls— did help out with specific tasks, including monitoring and tending, turning the care recipient in bed, flushing feeding tubes, and administering oxygen.

Prior divisions of household labor were also important, as they interfaced with skilled care work and in some cases had to be completely renegotiated.[12] For example, two husbands who provided care to their wives had different histories of doing housework. In one case, the couple had a traditional arrangement where he worked outside the home while she performed housework. Upon discovering she was ill, she taught him how to do the cooking and cleaning, so he learned how to do housework in addition to medical skills. In the other case, the husband had always performed some of the housework, and both he and his wife had worked outside the home, so the performance of additional housework or "support care" was not as new to him.

Even when there were similar divisions of labor in households, however, caregivers responded differently to their new duties. For example, three married couples caring for children had traditional arrangements where the wife was a full-time homemaker, or worked part time and had performed virtually all the housework, while the husband worked outside the home. Yet these couples negotiated their new work in different ways. In one case, the husband began taking over the shopping and the nighttime cooking while the wife performed the skilled care, and he eventually began performing some of the skilled work. They were finally able to obtain a waiver aide to help with some of the personal care. In the second case, the wife continued to take care of the regular housework and also performed all the skilled care. In the third, she continued to work part time and organized all of the skilled care, while he rotated the skilled work. Further studies on the specific variables that affect decision making in terms of housework and skilled medical care are needed. What is clear is that the introduction of skilled labor imposes additional constraints and causes caregivers to reflect critically on their unique situations and the particular resources that are available to them.[13] My interview subjects' preexisting work histories and divisions of labor coalesced with perceptions of available resources and informed a thought process for each caregiver: "What do I need to do?" and "What are my choices?"

This process caused individuals to prioritize the accomplishment of skilled labor over prior conceptions relating to unpaid and paid work. For example, Meredith said that she and her husband had quite egalitarian views, and although he performed much of the skilled work—"If I dropped dead today, he would be able to take care of my son"—they decided that she should stay home because of his better salary and benefits. For Isabelle and Randy, whose son had a brain injury, they agreed that she should stay home initially, but because her job had better benefits and it was easier for him to lift their son as he grew older and heavier, she eventually returned to work while he took a part-time job. Other caregivers carried out similar evaluations of their resources, and made lifestyle changes to accommodate care work. Some moved or changed jobs in order to fulfill caregiving needs. Annette, who cared for her mother, moved back home from another state in order to provide hands-on skilled care. Overall, what is apparent is that due to divisions of labor in homes, work patterns, and available resources, women are more likely to be in situations where they are giving skilled care *and* performing or organizing housework.

Moreover, prior studies have found that caregivers are reluctant to ask friends and family for help and may, as Abel (1991, 164) notes, "shield members of their networks from the consequences" of care work. This process seems especially pronounced in skilled care. Primary caregivers shoulder most tasks and tend to relinquish the skilled labor for very limited amounts of time, or give up only discrete pieces of the skilled procedures or other "unskilled" tasks. Because of the complexity and risk of skilled caregiving, there are fewer people they can turn to for help. Asking a friend or relative to babysit a child for an hour or two is entirely different from asking them to take care of a child who has a tracheostomy, and may exceed established bounds of reciprocity. Some caregivers said they did not want to make friends or other family members responsible for skilled care because they knew they would be afraid of hurting the care recipient, and said they understood when family members they cared for deeply did not feel that they could or should learn the procedures.

In some cases where other family members or close friends did perform specific procedures for a short time, it was mostly adult daughters, sisters, or sisters-in-law who helped on a limited basis during visits, or served as backup when caregivers were ill or had to work. This pattern supports prior work by Gerstel (2000), who maintains that women often engage in a "third shift" of labor (as compared to Hochschild and Machung's [1989] "second shift" of housework and childcare), whereby they take care of extended networks of family and friends.[14] The fact that it is women who tend to take on skilled medical labor for extended family members further adds to the multidimensional nature of unpaid labor that women perform.[15]

Caregivers also relied on women—sisters, daughters, sisters-in-law, and friends—for advice or emotional care, and to help with errands. Some also turned to family members or close friends who were professional nurses or caseworkers for advice, or for demonstrations of how to perform some of the labor. It is evident that women who are nurses or social workers are called on to give practical and professional help to their friends and family members who are facing a medical challenge. Thus, gender is evident in caregiving labor because of the position women have as caregivers in family life, and in professional work situations, where they are overrepresented in traditional caring occupations.[16]

Given the difficulty of negotiating paid work, unpaid housework, and child rearing, there is perhaps no greater caregiver strain than that faced by single parents or guardians. Although the number of children living with fathers has increased, women are much more likely to co-reside with children.[17] Single women who are caring for children are especially vulnerable to economic disadvantage in the labor market (Scott 2010) and may have to give up employment outside the home in order to provide care, as they may not have partners or other family members at home who are willing to share the skilled care.[18]

For three of the five single women (divorced, widowed, or separated) in this study who cared for children, marriages ended in separation or divorce because the women did not believe their husbands were able to contribute in a meaningful way to their caregiving duties. One woman told me that her ex-husband didn't do much when he was there and "slept all the time." Another said her husband became "jealous" of her care of her adult son. Of the five women, two had boyfriends or ex-husbands who performed some of the care and three had teenagers who helped. Four of these women did not work outside the home. One of the five had been laid off, and another fired from her job due to absence from work for caregiving. Three of the women reported injuries or medical disabilities that made caregiving, as well as working outside the home, more difficult. One caregiver was able to work full time due to the flexibility of her employer and her ability to work from home and the hospital on a computer. She also eventually qualified for waiver services, which allowed her to get help from a part-time nurse. Indeed, in all five of the cases, care recipients eventually received government help—four received waiver nurses, and two caregivers were eventually paid for some of their work through a state program. As noted in chapter 3, however, finding out about programs was often difficult and application processes were drawn out and full of snags. Also, while having a part-time nurse or government assistance helps, it does not replace income lost from full-time employment.

Further compounding women's care work is that they are more likely taking primary responsibility for multiple, sometimes simultaneous, caregiving roles—for example, caring for other children, family members with illnesses or disabilities, or the elderly.[19] Of the twenty-two women I interviewed, nineteen were in multiple caregiving roles part or all of the time they performed skilled labor. Sixteen were caring for other children, and three of these women had more than one child with disabilities or a chronic illness. Others were either directly caring or organizing care for their parents or other family members.

These multiple roles become especially problematic when the immediate need to perform medical procedures must take precedence over everything else. In these situations, caregivers simply cannot do two things at once or be in two places at one time. A caregiver described the stress of needing to be at a nursing home to oversee her mother's care while administering IV medications at home at noon:

> I got the air in the line and I'm just . . . I don't know what to do. And so I couldn't . . . do it. . . . So I called the home health nurse, and she says, 'Well I can't get there right now but I'll be there as soon as I can.' And I go, 'Okay.' . . . And . . . what I'm wanting to do is to get this done and go—get over to see—sign those papers. Well . . . it wasn't gonna work. She didn't get here till . . . about one. In the meantime, I called [the nursing home] and told them to forget it, 'cause I knew I wasn't gonna get out of here.

Although in some cases women had spouses to help out with child rearing, they were often worried when their multiple caregiving roles meant they could not provide the amount of care they wanted to for other children or relatives, or spend the amount of time with them that they would like. A mother whose child had a severe brain injury talked about her other son: "One thing . . . when I look back that I really regret is that I couldn't have spent more one-on-one time with him. He's turned out fabulous. But it's still—it's just like . . . that one thing that's always bothered me about it."

Importantly, good caregiving led some care recipients to be able to lead independent lives. Some finished college, began jobs, or later moved out on their own—in some cases with the help of government services. I spoke with six adult care recipients who were available at the time of the caregiver interviews and wanted to talk to me. They all expressed deep gratitude for what their caregivers had done. Grant said his mother helped him tremendously after his accident. "She knew what she had to do, and she did it," he said. "She's like, 'I know this is uncomfortable for you . . . but you gotta get it done.'"

Maintaining economic independence, however, could be challenging for care recipients. Marcus, who was living at home with his parents, was interviewing for jobs. Although he was thankful to have family support, he was frustrated that his disability income would not cover his monthly expenses. "Disability I get—five hundred bucks a month," he told me. "After paying a car payment and insurance, I got a hundred bucks for the month. It's not gonna work. I mean, I don't see how some people live off disability. I don't know how they *can*. Simply feeding yourself. . . . I don't know."

Indeed, the social safety net in the United States often does not provide enough for care recipients to maintain independence, and, as seen in chapter 3, they must also balance trying to work with maintaining insurance and other benefits.

As this chapter has demonstrated, analyzing "home" as a place of skilled care reveals many challenges, including geographical and physical limitations, coordination issues, intense self-evaluation processes by caregivers, and significant variations in milieu. Family formations, the division of household labor, care recipient independence, and economic considerations play prominent roles and influence the work that is done, and by whom. Economic resources are a crucial component, as most caregivers perform their work without pay or benefits and fall outside labor law protections, while many care recipients struggle to maintain independence. These challenges are invisible to a casual observer who may be far removed from the everyday labor processes necessary to maintain health. Opening a window to see inside multiple homes allows us to understand real needs, and gives us ideas about the policies needed to meet them.

5

"You Do What You Gotta Do"

Although it was very hard for me to give IVs to my own son, simply put, I believed I did it because I loved him, and I wanted him to be able to live as normal a life as possible. The medical professionals I worked with seemed very caring and told me that performing this work at home was something that most parents of children with such illnesses did. It seemed right to try to normalize this new work, and to help my son stay out of the hospital.

The feelings of wanting him to attend a good school, to have close friendships, and to be happy were all similar to the emotions I felt in assuming his care. His neighborhood, his room at home, and his friends were all important parts of his socialization. If the current expectation was that I should do this, then I would—after all, loving and caring for a child means that you do everything you can to help him.

So far I have talked mostly about caregivers' anxiety over the difficulties of the care work, but as prior scholars have noted, caregiving itself involves complex emotions and has rewards as well as burdens (Abel 1991, 59–68). According to England, Folbre, and Leana (2012, 23), although motivations to do care work may be *extrinsic*, including "expectation of direct payment or other rewards," "social approval," or even "postponed rewards such as reciprocity," they may also be *intrinsic*, such as "enjoyment of the . . . labor process itself." Relevant to family care work, these authors note that motivations may arise from a desire to contribute to the happiness or well-being of a specific person—the "form of altruism most commonly identified as love" (24). In reality, they say, "a mix of motivational forms" may be at play, such as genuine care, taken-for-granted norms about gender roles, and societal approval (24).

It is important to remember that these motivations—even those fueled by love—do not erase social structural constraints like those discussed in chapter 3, but rather call us to recognize human feelings as they exist in relationships within social structure. Doing so allows us to better understand not only those who feel genuine care, but those who may not.[1]

Importantly, the caregivers I interviewed for this book all spoke very positively of their relationships with care recipients, and it was apparent that they had deep emotional investments, which had often developed over many months or years before skilled care was needed. When talking about their labor, they seamlessly integrated their feelings of love and care with the labor processes they enacted. They shared with me their notes, medicine charts, humorous cartoons they used to cope, timelines, diaries, and favorite pictures. The fact that caregivers agreed to be interviewed speaks clearly as to their investment in the labor, and their perceptions of its importance.

This chapter examines the complexity of caregivers' feelings about the labor they perform; it probes their emotions and their identities. How do they frame and make sense of the labor they perform? How are their perspectives tied to their identities? I ask these questions within the framework of prior studies of emotion work and emotional labor and Erickson and Stacey's (2013) theory of *emotion practice*, which advocates considering both macro- and microprocesses, as well as context, in examining the emotional labor of both paid and unpaid workers. I also take insights from Lopez's (2006) *organized emotional care*, which demonstrates how structural supports have been instrumental in reducing the emotional burdens of paid care workers in institutional settings. The analyses of emotion and identity for caregivers and nurses alike are seen within the context of the mutual labor process that is enacted—a labor process that transfers professional skills from paid to unpaid workers (see Glazer 1993).

Emotion Work and Emotional Labor

It is impossible to adequately analyze the emotionality of caregivers, and also nurses, without drawing on past scholarship in emotion at home and at work—venues where, scholars have argued, feelings of identity and emotions are paramount (Burawoy 1979; Hochschild 1983, 2003). The seminal concepts on the role of emotion and identity at home and in paid work are Hochschild's (1983, 2003) *emotion work* (occurring in private, at-home contexts), and *emotional labor* (occurring in workplaces).

In regard to private emotion work, Hochschild maintains that society's "feeling rules" dictate how we think we *should* feel. For example, we are supposed to cry at funerals. Hochschild gives numerous examples of occasions when people work hard on their emotions and use "deep acting" to make themselves feel in ways they think they should feel. "We must dwell on what we want to feel and on what we must do to induce the feeling," she states (2003, 47). People may psych themselves up, or even "lie to themselves" (46), in order to try to change feelings. These matters need "constant attention, continual question, and testing" (42) and are done for the "pursuit of fulfillment . . . in everyday life" (55).

Based on her study of the emotional processes used by flight attendants, Hochschild (2003, 119) describes emotional labor as occurring in workplaces where employees must manage emotion in order to comply with company feeling rules. Flight attendants are supposed to smile and put the customer first, even when they don't feel like it. Hochschild (14) argues that when emotions are used for the pursuit of profit, they become commodified. She fashions this type of emotional labor as exploitative, particularly if workers engage in deep acting in order to change their feelings to comply with company feeling rules. In this process, workers experience a loss of identity (135–36).

The concept of emotional labor has been widely used by workplace sociologists to understand identity processes for paid service and care workers, and has expanded greatly since Hochschild's (1983) work. Workplace sociologists have critiqued and broadened the concept, finding that workers' coping mechanisms, the work environment itself, and the positive rewards of their jobs mean that workers who perform emotional labor do not always suffer a loss of self in the course of labor processes (Tolich 1993; Bolton and Boyd 2003; Lopez 2006, 2010; Stacey 2011). Sharon

Bolton, who has extensively studied nurses' emotional labor and identity, finds that nurses have multifaceted forms of emotional labor and are skilled "emotional jugglers" who are able to adapt to the situation at hand without experiencing negative impacts on their identity (2001).[2] In her work with Boyd (2003), she critiques Hochschild's notion that emotional work is always done for the good of the company, and depicts four separate categories of emotional labor: *pecuniary* (in response to commercial demands), *prescriptive* (in response to professional demands), *presentational* ("the basic socialized self"), and *philanthropic* (giving emotions as "gifts") (295–97). Bolton and Boyd see philanthropic emotional labor or authentic relationships as possible and taking place in private "unmanaged spaces"—free from employer mandates (303).

The very way in which work is structurally organized has also been studied by workplace and care work scholars in terms of the impact on work processes and emotional labor. Prior scholarship has demonstrated that institutions typically present time challenges for care workers who are trying to complete tasks, and that time for emotional care may be limited (Diamond 1992; Foner 1994; Chambliss 1996; Lopez 2004; 2006). In his study of nursing aides working in institutional settings, Lopez (2006) found that workplaces that practice "organized emotional care" prioritize relationships between staff and patients by providing more space for authentic interactions to occur. In these workplaces, feelings of exploitation from emotional labor can give way to spaces were relationships have more room to flourish. Scholars have also focused on care work at the job level: for example, England, Folbre, and Leana (2012, 22) argue that the strategic redesign of care jobs can improve intrinsic motivation for care workers. Scholars have pointed out that the context of the work matters greatly. Erickson and Stacey (2013, 182) argue that typical workplace feeling rules cannot be applied to all care work jobs. Telling a customer to "have a nice day," they argue, is much different from the emotional skills needed to take care of terminally ill patients and their families.

Indeed, the context in which a particular occupation occurs has great consequences for the performance of emotional labor. Grandey, Diefendorff, and Rupp (2013) discuss some occupations or roles that have "fuzzy boundaries" regarding their classification as emotional labor (associated with paid work) or emotion work (associated with unpaid work).[3] For example, they argue that there is a gray area for home health aides because although the workers receive a wage, frequently interact with the public, and have emotion performance as part of their role requirement, they are also operating in a private context—the home (Grandey, Diefendorff, and Rupp 2013, 19). Stacey (2005, 2011) explores these dynamics in her study of home care aides and finds that they face multiple contradictions. Although they must draw appropriate boundaries, they are considered "fictive kin," (2011, 102) and find deep meaning in their care work.

While Stacey's work is important in that it examines emotional labor by paid care workers in the home, workplace scholars have not generally examined the emotion work of family caregivers who are performing skilled medical labor. In regard to family caregivers, Grandey, Diefendorff, and Rupp (2013, 19) note that even though emotion performance may be a role requirement, the work would likely be considered not emotional labor but emotion work, because it is done in a private setting, is not linked to financial gains, and lacks frequent interactions with the public, and because management does not monitor and evaluate the emotional performance.

I argue that the "fuzzy boundaries" that occur when paid workers perform labor in the context of a private home also occur when family caregivers are executing skilled nursing tasks—tasks that are far outside typical household labor, and are learned from paid professionals. Family caregivers *do* have paid supervisors monitoring and evaluating their work, and their emotions are evaluated by home health nurses, as in cases in which their attitudes toward care recipients are not deemed caring enough. They are also often responsible for interacting with various outside agencies and vendors in implementing their work.

These complications in how to adequately describe this labor and its emotional components are exactly what care work scholars recognize in their call to more fully integrate the study of labor processes across paid and unpaid boundaries (see, for example, Folbre and Wright 2012; Erickson and Stacey 2013). Hochschild's dichotomies of emotion work and emotional labor are indeed blurred in shared labor processes that involve both paid and unpaid workers.

Drawing on Bourdieu's (1977, 1990a, 1990b) general theory of practice, Erickson and Stacey (2013, 175–80) have advocated *emotion practice* as a theoretical framework that melds the care work and emotional labor literatures, recognizes the nature of care work as distinctly different from other types of jobs due to the high expectation of caring and the centrality of physical labor (Theodosius 2008), sees context as key, and considers both micro- and macrolevels of analysis. The authors also urge scholars to consider occupational context in their studies of emotional labor, as well as the structural and power differences at play in interactions (Erickson and Stacey 2013, 179–80).

In this vein, I argue that we must begin to recognize and study the emotion work/emotional labor link between unpaid caregivers and paid professionals if we are to ever understand the underlying work processes in home health care. In performing this analysis, I concentrate next on emotion work and identity for caregivers—sticking to Hochschild's original terms for clarity, and drawing on past literature that analyzes emotion work in the home. In the next chapter I focus on caregiver interactions with medical professionals and the emotional labor and identities of home health nurses, paying attention to key features of the work process such as context and occupational identity. All are important elements of the skilled labor transfer.

Identity, Relationships, and Skilled Caregiving

In unpacking the emotion work/emotional labor link within the context of an emotion practice framework, I first consider the work of feminist and family scholars who have studied emotion work in the home (Daniels 1987; DeVault 1991, Mac Rae 1998). According to Lively (2013, 233), much of the prior scholarship has focused on the emotion management strategies of individuals and their emotional investments in family members, especially children. Prior studies have demonstrated that women are much more likely to carry out this work—which involves attending to emotional needs and informal types of caregiving—than are men (Hochschild with Machung 1989; Lively 2013, 233). Some sociologists have examined the link between emotion work and perceived inequities in household labor (Lively, Steelman, and Powell 2010) and the ways in which these perceived inequities are negotiated (Hochschild with Machung 1989). Hochschild finds that some couples deal with negative emotions by adopting "family myths" that gloss over inequities and recast their situations in a more positive light (Hochschild with Machung 1989, 19; Lively 2013, 233).

In regard to emotion work and family caregiving, Mac Rae's (1998) study sheds light on the emotion management used by family caregivers of Alzheimer's patients (many of whom had changed personalities). Caregivers felt guilty when they violated feeling rules and couldn't manage their emotions. They felt bad when they did not feel they loved the care recipient in the way that they should, and some felt guilty about being resentful (144–45). According to Mac Rae, those who engaged in this type of self-process were in danger of being alienated from their true feelings and suffering a loss of self.[4]

Emotion work has also been analyzed not just as a management of feeling rules—where individuals work on their emotions and feel guilty if they do not feel the way they think they should—but, to quote James (1989, 21), as a "social process" that involves "dealing with other people's feelings."[5] James embeds her definition in the socialist feminist view that emotion work is "hard work" that is performed for others at home and at work, is often invisible, and aids in social reproduction. She states that emotion work involves "juggling," responding, and engaging in active listening (26–27).

Similarly, Daniels (1987, 409), referring to Hochschild's (1979) "positive aspects of 'emotion work,'" gives examples of activities that emphasize taking care of the emotional well-being of others—for example, "attending carefully to how a setting affects others in it—through taking the role of the other and feeling some of the same feelings." Both Daniels and James maintain that emotion work is often invisible and that women fail to see it as work.

In a similar vein, Erickson (1993, 2005), drawing on Hochschild (1979) and Thoits (1996), also operationalizes emotion work as actively managing others' feelings. In referring to Hochschild, she states that "within a personal or familial context, this work tends to involve the enhancement of others' emotional well-being and the provision of emotional support" (Erickson 1993, 888). Erickson sees emotion work as an active and agentic part of women's construction of gender identity (Erickson 2005). She discusses the implications of gender construction theory, in that the emotion work women do is not perceived as alienating, but rather shows their concern for family members, and is used to construct their gender identity as a positive part of selfhood (Erickson 2005, 340).

As we have seen, emotion work in the home, then, has been constructed to mean working on one's own feelings as well as actively managing the feelings of others (Hochschild 1983; James 1989; Daniels 1987; Erickson 1993, 2005). This concept of emotion work as active also has support within the sociology of work, where multiple scholars have made the case that workers do not always experience emotional labor in negative, passive ways that cause alienation (Tolich 1993; Bolton 2000, 2001; Bolton and Boyd 2003; Lopez 2006; Stacey 2011). Emotional labor in the workplace—particularly in health care settings, where care is expected (Erickson and Stacey 2013), as well as at home—takes negotiation, action, interaction, and giving time to others (James 1989). In the private and public (paid work) spheres, emotion work and emotional labor, respectively, can be seen as both "feeling" and "doing" (see Erickson 2011). As we will see, both are critical to the emotion work/emotional labor link performed in skilled care work.

Identity in Relationships

Family caregiving begins in relationships (Glenn 2000; Abel 1991) and, according to Glenn (2010, 187), is an interdependent process, in which both caregiver and care recipient have power. Indeed, the caregivers in this book incorporated skilled caregiving into their existing relationships and identities as mother, father, spouse, child (see also Heaton 1999). This process is evident in the story of Alice, who told me about her strong desire to take care of her adult daughter, even against the advice of medical professionals, who recommended a nursing home. "No," she said, "I just . . . brought her home with me, and was up in the middle of the night just like she was a baby and took care of her . . . and did what I had to do."

In my analysis of caregivers' identities and emotionality, many of the caregivers demonstrated what England, Folbre, and Leana (2012, 23) refer to as "prosocial intrinsic motives." Evidence of genuine feelings of caring for care recipients was prominent. Some caregivers described special events and parties they planned so that their loved ones could share family time. Many relayed moments of warmth and humor. Sidney talked about how, when his wife became unable to communicate before she passed away, he listened to her through the use of a transparent alphabet. "You'd hold it up and she would look at the letter, and . . . you just watch her eyes spell out what she wanted to spell," he said. In trying to convey that she felt "claustrophobic," she misspelled the word. "What the hell starts with klos?" he asked her, and it became a joke for them.

Because such preexisting relationships exist prior to the enactment of medical skills, the identity component in the work process is vastly different from that for paid workers. In Burawoy's (1979) study, workers' identities were formed from workplace relations, and in Sherman's (2007) analysis, identities at work were only tempered by preexisting identities. Family caregivers' unique preexisting relationships with care recipients set them apart, even from paid care workers who are performing work in the home (for example, see Stacey 2011). Understanding the centrality of relationship provides unique perspectives into emotion work and problematizes the assumption of alienation implicit in purely structural views of the labor process.[6]

All the caregivers I interviewed spoke of the care work process as a top priority in their lives. Regarding his wife's wound care, Paul told me, "You make a decision. Is this my life or is my life still global?" If you "*can* do these things," you do them, he said, and he listened when his wife stated to him, "I'd rather you do these things than anyone else." As would be expected, in cases of spouses, some caregivers spoke of reciprocity in the relationship. Sidney told me, "People will say, . . . 'You're so wonderful to do this,' . . . and it's like, 'What are you talking about?' This is just what you do. You just assume that if the shoe were on the other foot, that she would do the same thing for me."[7] Bill explained that when he brought his dying nephew home to live with him, the two had long had an extremely close relationship. "He asked me to bring him home . . . because he so much enjoyed my place, and there's no way that I was going to say no, that you can't come to my place to pass," he said.

As we have seen, caregivers framed their labor in terms of the relationship and their loved ones' immediate needs, which demanded an active response. They spoke with intensity about how they used technology and skilled procedures to feed, bandage, give lifesaving medications, and suction and provide oxygen to care recipients so they could breathe.

Caregivers wanted care recipients to be comfortable, normal, and healthy, and saw them as "whole people"—people to whom they afforded dignity and love (Abel 1991, 76–79; also see Kittay 1999).

"Doing What You Gotta Do": Emotion Work and Interactions with Care Recipients

The caregivers I interviewed clearly engaged in emotion work in managing their own emotions as well as those of care recipients. A few spoke about the need to stay positive, even if they were not feeling well themselves. In talking about how she gives support to her husband, Barbara said it is important to "just try to be encouraging and try not to express your anxieties, if you're having a bad day as a caregiver. Don't necessarily say words like, 'I wish I didn't sign up for this,' you know? I've never said that and I would never say that, but some people do and I think that's wrong because I think that hurts the patient's emotional stability and it also hurts the relationship."

In managing their own feelings and insecurities about the labor, caregivers often pushed back their own emotions. "I just stepped up" or "I sucked it up and did it" were typical responses. Some expressed that they initially wished that a qualified person could do the labor. Many caregivers said they pushed out negative thoughts. Beverly told me, "I kind of built up my confidence and tried not to think too much about it. It had to be done and I had to do it." Bridget said that questions like "What if I make him sick? What if he *died*?" ran through her mind. But, she said, "you can't dwell on it, or else you'd never get nothing done." Indeed, some caregivers said they were so busy that they "didn't have time to think about anything else." These processes lead us to question the structural limitations that are imposed on caregivers, such as payer guidelines that limit nurses' visits (see chapter 3). In this regard, alternative systems that assure adequate time for caregivers to learn and provide needed support—essentially incorporating Lopez's (2006) organized emotional care—would be highly beneficial for caregivers and care recipients alike.

Caregivers also managed the emotions of care recipients. They talked about trying to cheer them up or give emotional support, and took active measures to express concern when they knew care recipients were in pain or were afraid. Adrienne said, about her son, "You don't know from one day to the next . . . how he's gonna get up [in the morning]. . . . When I walk in there, [I say,] 'Hi, handsome,' you know? . . . I mean he's always happy but then you could see that there's pain. You can see the pain in the eyes."

These instances of emotional encouragement sometimes occurred during intense periods of stress when caregivers had to reassure care recipients or calm them down. In some cases, caregivers monitored the amount of information they gave to care recipients to keep them from worrying. A husband who took care of his wife told me about a time when he discovered that the bottom of her foot "had a green and black area on it that was *terrible* looking. . . . She's very squeamish about some things—blood . . . and things going on in her body—so I knew not to really go into detail." As he processed this new and potentially unnerving sight, he told his wife that there was a problem, helped her get dressed, and rushed her to the ER.

In other cases, care recipients were well aware there was a problem. A mother told me that at times her son would experience spasms that constricted his chest, and this would set off a panic attack. "Sometimes it would last for forty-five minutes," she said, during which she would "either be using the cough machine . . . or an Ambu bag." During his screams of "I'm gonna die!" she would try to coach him through his anxiety.

It is interesting to contrast these caregivers' emotions and actions—feeling and doing—with prior conceptualizations of emotion work. In Mac Rae's work, caregivers had feelings that were at odds with cultural norms. They believed, for example, that they "shouldn't feel" resentment (Mac Rae 1998, 144–45). The caregivers I interviewed indeed had feelings that ran counter to cultural norms, but in different ways. Although a few did express guilt about their feelings—as one said, "I think it's a burden, I mean, I hate to say that but it's always on my mind"—for the most part caregivers did not so much express feelings of guilt as worry about the potential of *doing* something wrong, or not *doing* enough.

An issue for many of the caregivers was the disjuncture between general cultural feeling rules, which guide the expectations of individuals' roles—for example, as parents, children, or spouses—and the reality of their immediate situation, which demanded an active response of doing skilled labor. In this context, cultural feeling rules appear vague. We "take care of" each other when we are sick. We want to "be a good mother, spouse, child." But cultural feeling rules don't capture the enormity and complexity of what needs to be *done* in skilled work. Caregivers were, to borrow from Smith (1987, 49), on a fault line between cultural expectations and reality.

What was common to the caregivers I interviewed was that—despite feelings of disjuncture between cultural feeling rules and the realities they observed—a sense of needing to *do* trumped their anxiety over learning and executing new skills. In contrast, then, to those who "work on their feelings" to make themselves *feel* the way they should, skilled labor caregivers managed their feelings and worked up to *doing*. Consequently, they were not left to stew about an appropriate response—"Should I do this or that?"—but instead focused on action. After all, they had medical actors telling them what is necessary to do, so what needed to be done was not really open for judgment. Thus, the most common way caregivers described their feelings was that the labor is something you "have to do": "You do what you gotta do." "I just gotta do what I gotta do to keep her well." "I don't really view it as a duty or a chore. I just do what I have to do." "I don't know, coping, you don't think about it at the time. So it's just what you *do*."[8] While these responses are made within the context of social structure—which in many cases lacks viable alternatives and structural support for the labor—they are also made within the context of preexisting relationships, ones that encompass human feelings, interactions, identities, and needs.

In this regard, caregivers' concern was squarely for the health and well-being of care recipients. Paul's case demonstrates how caregivers were somehow able to mentally mesh their concern for their loved one with the procedures they enacted. When I asked him how he felt the first time he realized what he would have to do, he stated,

> I gotta do it. . . . There was no question in my mind that, "Well, why do I have to do it? Why can't you have someone come and do it?" . . . Well no . . . she's the light of my life. And then there was . . . the two drains and then there was a hole in her chest here. And that is because the incision had not knitted correctly up here. And so it started out as three times a day. . . . I had to pull out the packing that was in there, and then I went and took some sterile gauze and cut a strip about that wide and that long. . . . I took

a long Q-tip, a swab, and I had to poke it in there until it was packed completely. And then cover it with . . . a piece of gauze taped over the top and then put a four-by-four [bandage] on top of that.

Prior research has shown that caregivers also seek to increase positive identity for care recipients.[9] As part of "feeling and doing," caregivers in this study said they considered not only the physical effects of procedures on loved ones, but also the effects on their emotional well-being and identity. For example, a mother who takes care of a suprapubic catheter not only talked about the procedures she performs, but also said she tries to consider her son's feelings when going to school with a urinary catheter: "It's not on his leg, it's got a real long hose so I can hang it, like, from the edge of the chair and get it out of the way where it's not—where he can go to school and not be embarrassed 'cause he's carrying pee around with him."

Thus, the centrality of relationship drives the way in which physical labor is enacted, and caregivers manage not only their own emotions, but the emotions and well-being of care recipients as well.

Identity in Work, Love, and Life

The emotion work and actions of caregivers, their feeling and doing, caused many changes—in their perceptions of their work, and in their interactions with others. Oftentimes, friends and acquaintances could not fully grasp what they were doing.[10] A mom told me, "We don't really complain about anything, so people at work don't really . . . understand what we do. . . . They just don't . . . because we don't claim it. . . . We had some friends . . . [say], 'Let's go out of town and spend the weekend.' . . . They just don't think about it." A few also said it is sometimes hard when they hear others complain—for example, if coworkers complain about overtime, or if friends complain about what caregivers perceive as comparatively trivial issues. A mother whose child suffered a brain injury after an accident told me, "We just live differently than if it hadn't happened. It . . . put things into perspective. . . . If someone's complaining they had a really rough day doing something . . . I just think, 'No, that's not rough compared to what it could be.' "

Corbin and Strauss (1988, 289) found that caregivers of spouses with chronic illnesses often don't want to talk about the issues they face because they don't want to be considered " 'bad' spouses." In studying adult-daughter caregivers of Alzheimer's patients, Abel (1991, 113) found that "because their own notions of good care compel them to camouflage their activities, they discourage rather than invite gratitude," and thus seldom "receive the affirmation they seek." "Camouflaging" activities becomes harder in skilled care. Therefore, even though caregivers may not speak a great deal about their labor to coworkers or acquaintances, extended family members and close friends often know of the work that is done. Meredith told me that when her mom visits, she tells Meredith, "I don't think you understand what you guys *do* every day and what it looks like."

In this regard, it is notable that in describing their labor, the caregivers I interviewed generally did not downplay the work they did, and fully acknowledged the amount of time and skill their labor takes.[11] A mother described the labor as "a second full-time job," and another caregiver commented that going home from work still brings "another eight hours" of "work" to do. Yet even though caregivers sometimes described their labor as "work" or a "job," as noted earlier (and by Heaton 1999), caregivers formed their thoughts about their caregiving labor within the context of the relationship.[12] The following quote, from a wife who was let go from her job due to the amount of time that was necessary for care work, demonstrates the simultaneous recognition of the scope of work and of the feelings about it: "There were a lot of times I viewed it as work. It was my full-time job. And it was the hardest work I ever did. But I also viewed it as an act of love, because we took our wedding vows seriously and I promised him that we would be together till he died. And he used to get so upset and I'd say, 'If it was me, would you do it?' 'Well of *course* I would.' And I said, 'So what's the difference?'"

The daily work processes and interactions of caregivers, however, serve to create and reiterate cultural differences between self and others. Newfound working knowledge means that caregivers learn to speak a different language—one that appears highly medicalized to others. Marcie, a mom, told me that although she had no medical background, "everyone teases me now that I do": "Sometimes when I talk to my family and friends . . . they're like, 'What?' [*Laughs.*] I think that I'm talking . . . very common terms, and they look at me like, 'What are you talking about?'"

These cultural adaptations occur not only in the use of language but, as we have seen, in the operation of technological instruments and objects such as pumps and devices. Ogburn (1922, 200) posited that when material culture (in this case medical equipment) changes, there is a period of "cultural lag" where people must come to terms with the nonmaterial culture—such as norms of behavior—surrounding the change. Thus, while caregivers incorporate skilled care into their preexisting identities, they must also respond to new role requirements within their status of "mother," "father," "child." Caregivers indeed feel and do things differently from those around them. They also undergo significant life challenges and must negotiate the nuances of their preexisting relationships with loved ones. Hannah fears that if something ever happened to her or her husband, they might have to place her son, who has both cognitive impairments and skilled medical needs, in an institution. She said, "Those are [the] kind of decisions that most parents are probably not making— that kind of future plans for their kids . . . but we're kind of forced to . . . and . . . it kind of upsets us."

Considering the changes caregivers undergo and the intense emotionality, they identified both positive and negative effects of the emotional and physical labor on their identities. As we have seen, caregivers said they "sucked it up and did it." Some believed the labor had made them "harder" or "stronger." A wife who cares for her husband commented, "I think it has made me a harder person because I don't take much flak from anybody. So I have to keep that in check. . . . And sometimes it's hard for me to do. Because I . . . know what I want and what I need. . . . And I don't stop till I get there. . . . And before—I probably—I *know* I wasn't that way, because I wasn't raised to be that way."

The relationship thus spurs caregivers to do what they can for those they care about, with the resulting labor process creating many changes. Importantly, although caregivers acknowledged the difficult aspects of the labor—lack of sleep, worry, and anxiety—they also seemed to derive emotional benefits from knowing that they helped those they loved.[13] Bridget told me, "I'm glad I was able to do it. . . . Makes me feel better, knowing that I was able to help him." And Cheryl said, "Makes me feel like there are tools out there that we can use to contribute to her health." Caregivers also took pride in the quality of care they believed they provided. "He never had any skin breakdown. . . . He stayed well hydrated, well nourished," said one. And a mother, speaking of bowel and urinary functions, told me, "He never had an accident."[14]

When I asked Marcie if doing home care affected the way she feels about herself, her answer reflected her strong feelings for her children and her view that her skilled labor has helped them: "I think maybe [it's] made me feel important. . . . I mean my whole life has been the kids . . . so I think [about] . . . what I can do to help *them*. . . . I don't really view it as a duty or a chore. . . . I just do what I have to do. . . . No—it's not something I would pick. . . . I wouldn't sit down [and think I'd] . . . *want* to do this. But if I *can* do it and it helps them, and they need it, then I do it." Several caregivers also found that the situation had put things in perspective, that their religious faith had grown, or that they no longer worried about small things.[15] Said Nancy, "I mellowed big time. . . . I don't worry about little things. I was always [a] very immaculate person with the house, and everything had to be just right . . .—that's very unimportant. Material things don't mean anything to me . . . you know, like they did."

Many expressed that they have more empathy for others. Sidney said,

> Certain things that you . . . *do* think about . . . were life changes. I don't believe in right or wrong anymore. There's no right, if somebody wants a trach and somebody else doesn't, there is no right or wrong choice there. . . . Somebody does something to help the person they're taking care of, and . . . [they make] a mistake, it turns out one way or another, they aren't wrong. I wouldn't call myself a flaming liberal by any stretch, but I think I probably have [a] more liberal or open view of life and other people now . . . because of the stuff that we [my wife and I] went through together.

Some caregivers said the situation had made family members, including children, more compassionate, or they felt that the way they handled things had been a positive example to other people. Several said they experienced more quality time with the care recipient and other family members. Some also said it changed their outside relationships—friends who couldn't handle the situation fell away, and other friends became closer. In regard to marriages, as seen in chapter 4, there were situations where husbands could not handle the care work for children; however, there were also situations where couples became closer. Meredith told me, "I think my husband and I—going through it together . . . that made us have a much more intimate relationship than I think anything could have—ever . . . because we went through it together and we came out of it stronger. So I think that really helps. . . . He and I can talk to each other."

Some caregivers said their new skills made them feel more confident. One caregiver said she realized "we can do anything that we need to." Ava, who originally felt very disinclined toward nursing, said, "It has made me more confident. I am a wimp. . . . And to know what I have done for him . . . he can't believe, you know."[16]

Notably, while caregivers recounted many positive effects of the labor on their relationships and their identities, their experiences could also have negative effects. Because caregivers prioritize care recipients' health, obviously there are intense periods when they feel anxiety and continue to push themselves. According to Adrienne, "It does get—the burden is heavy. But you just get up and you keep going and going. And . . . I have never crashed . . . from it, mentally or anything, because I know he needs me." And a single mom stated, "There was times when I was like, 'Okay, I'm done. I can't do no more. . . . I give up.' But then I never could do it. I couldn't do it. I couldn't let somebody else take care of my kid."

As seen in previous chapters, some caregivers experienced being unable to work or were fired from jobs due to caregiving duties. A single mom who hurt her back lifting her son told me it was "impossible" to work outside the home. "Between doctors' appointments and therapies . . . it's plain impossible," she said.

These experiences not only diminish resources, but also curb activities that could have positive effects on identity. As seen in prior research,[17] as well as my own, caregivers often give up time for leisure and relaxation. Some talk about how it is hard to travel or take vacations. In these ways, there is a danger of caregivers becoming inward focused or missing out on experiences in which they might grow in other ways. As a caregiver told me, "I just, I think that I'm becoming more secluded. . . . I think I'm just tired and when I had all the energy before to really put into calling family and calling friends . . . I think I'm just kind of a little bit more wore out."

Because caregivers "do what they gotta do," it is extremely hard for them to self-limit the care they give. Bounds of relationships are endless and are not dictated by time clocks. There is a danger of caregivers' own needs going unmet while they focus on the needs of care recipients. Those who care might also do labor despite their reluctance, and/or may feel that they can never do enough.

In this regard, nursing scholars Day and Anderson (2011) posit that compassion fatigue—a concept that has long been applied to occupations such as victims' advocates who assist those who have experienced trauma (Doerner and Lab 2015, 130)—may also apply to informal caregivers. The authors note that compassion fatigue may include feelings of burnout and negative emotions such as helplessness, or the inability to empathize (Day and Anderson 2011, 2). Although their work focuses primarily on caregivers of dementia patients, these effects can also have ramifications for caregivers performing nursing procedures. We need to understand more about the long-term consequences for caregivers who "step it up" to provide skilled care and strive to balance this complex new work and its emotional components.

As seen in chapter 3, it is also important to understand how social structural policies and the mix of payer sources set guidelines and limits on caregivers' work. As this chapter has shown, understanding more about the emotion work that caregivers do within these limits is vital. "You do what you gotta do" expresses both feeling and doing in care work, which can lead to positive identity and deeper relationships, but the phrase also sums up the costs and constraints of caregiving.

Indeed, the emotional and interactional components of care work are foundational to our understanding of the care labor process, yet they are not currently considered in U.S. health policy (see chapter 3). How appropriate if the lessons learned in institutions—lessons in how organized emotional care (Lopez 2006) can be applied to reduce the emotional labor of paid care workers—could be applied to caregivers who are practicing skilled medical labor in private homes, which lack labor law protections such as minimum wages, child labor limits, and FMLA. Policies that value caregivers' work and commitment, and mandate that they have enough time not only to learn and incorporate procedures but to practice emotional care, including self-care, would be highly beneficial.

6

Work Shifts

My husband, my mother-in-law, and I often took turns in overnight hospital stays when my son was young. We slept on a cot—actually, it was a chair that let out. It always hurt our backs, so we would come up with adaptations. An extra blanket or two rolled under our necks, a pillow propped under the small of our backs. We discussed strategies. When to take showers? Which residents were on call and when would they be rounding? I always hoped it was the funny one, or the one who was particularly kind. These conversations were important. They added some structure and knowledge to our common experiences. Usually we had slept little, knowing that at all times we would be the first to hear the beeping of IV poles and various alarms. How was the oxygen level? Was everything all right?

In thinking back on these times, I often felt that I was "on watch"—there to protect my son and ask the right questions, to communicate if I sensed a problem. The identities and emotion work of caregivers indeed frame their interactions with medical professionals. Many of the caregivers I interviewed shared similar experiences and feelings. They also said they spoke up when they witnessed situations that made them uneasy, such as the improper administration of procedures, or failures in protocol. Previous scholarship bears out these accounts and shows that caregivers are often extremely vigilant and protective when their loved ones are in institutional settings (Foner 1994; Bowers 1990). They may worry about a shortage of staff, or the potential for mistakes, and stay for long periods of time to perform much of the care work themselves (Lindhardt, Bolmsjö, and Hallberg 2006, 143).

As we have seen, interactions in institutions are paramount in setting the tone for at-home work processes (see chapter 2), yet much more needs to be known about caregivers' interactions with medical professionals at home. Clearly, in their evolving roles as skilled care workers, caregivers develop an intricate and heightened awareness of their loved ones' physical and emotional needs.[1] But how does this play out in labor processes at home, particularly in relationships with home health nurses and other medical professionals on whom caregivers depend? In the context of the home, emotional labor boundaries between paid and unpaid workers are murky (Stacey 2005, 2011; Grandey, Diefendorff, and Rupp 2013), and understanding the power dynamics—which have not often been studied in regard to emotional labor (Erickson and Stacey 2013)—is critical.

In this chapter, I take a closer look at these caregiver/nurse interactions. I include an analysis of the identities and emotional labor of home health nurses. As professionals who possess valuable disciplinary knowledge, how do they feel about transferring their skills to lay caregivers? Nurses' orientation to the labor and the effects on interactions with caregivers are key features in the labor transfer.

Relationships with Home Health Nurses

Because of caregivers' vigilance and their large emotional investments in care recipients' physical and emotional health, they have high expectations that medical personnel will display not only competency, but also caring attitudes toward their loved ones (see Abel 1991, 143). Much of the prior work on family relationships with home health providers has focused on relationships with home health aides. In semistructured interviews with both family members and their aides, Piercy and Woolley (1999,1) found that "good quality care" was described as being able to perform essential tasks, as well as having good relational skills. Piercy and Dunkley (2004, 175) found that caregivers of the elderly felt that "good quality paid home care" promoted quality of life for care recipients and resulted in "improved perceptions of their performances as caregivers." On the other hand, the authors note, "when paid home care was of poor quality, caregivers felt more stress and increased their monitoring of providers."

As providers of care who are dependent on medical professionals, caregivers inhabit a vulnerable position,[2] one that is exacerbated by social structural variables such as payer mixes, and also by inequalities in gender, race, and class (Meyer, Herd, and Michel 2000; Malat and Hamilton 2006). Kittay (1999, 14) argues that society fails to recognize that those who care for others face systematic inequalities because of their deeply embedded connections to those who need care. Thus, understanding the relative power of caregivers is important.

The medical establishment often uses surveys as a way to gauge satisfaction with services. Yet prior studies in which patients are interviewed have shown that high rates of satisfaction on health experience surveys actually hide a number of negative experiences (Williams, Coyle, and Healy 1998). Edwards, Staniszweska, and Crichton (2004, 168) found that patients may be reluctant to give negative evaluations due to their position of relative dependency in the health care system, their perceived need to maintain a positive relationship with care providers, and their desire to keep up a positive outlook in general.

The caregivers in this book were encouraged to speak freely about their interactions in order to capture both positive and negative experiences. Importantly, the majority generally described good relationships with individual nurses. As would be expected, when nurses or medical personnel showed caring or concern, caregivers expressed gratitude and trust. Caregivers valued nurses who adequately explained procedures and allowed time for understanding. Barbara described a home health nurse's positive interaction with her children and husband: "She's always happy, she's always encouraging, she interacts with our kids, she allows them to stay and visualize and to understand what she's doing."

The caregivers I interviewed were encouraged when nurses prioritized not only the physical but also the emotional well-being of care recipients, and when they recognized them as individuals who had a life outside of medical care. Phoebe described what she liked about a nurse who was eventually assigned through a waiver program (which allows nurses to stay for longer periods of time than those who are simply there to teach). The nurse asked about her son's feelings and what he liked to do:

> Well [at] first I was really nervous . . . having somebody else come in and take care of my kid that's never even seen my kid before. But she . . . asked the right questions. . . . "When does he take his pills? And when does he get cathed? And when does he—does he like to play games? *Can* he play games?" 'Cause that's my son, his whole life is games . . . and they would sit down in his room and she would watch him play that game and comment on it, and . . . just basically give him a hard time like I would. And I liked that.

Notably, although interactions with nurses were generally positive, caregivers also described several situations where there were issues—either in agencies' lack of response or in attitudes of staff. According to a wife, "It is unsettling when someone comes into our home . . . where they act like they don't want to be there." And a mom told me that when nurses come to check on her son, "they're always in a hurry," and she believes they rely too much on her to monitor his care. She said, "He's my son and I think that everybody should look over every square inch of him . . .—that's what I do. And I guess it's probably because I do it all the time, that they don't feel like they have to, you know?"

The mandates of payer sources and/or nurses' workloads may contribute to nurses feeling rushed in these situations. As we have seen, the structure of the labor process—where nurses have limited time and depend on caregiver labor—can place excess burdens on caregivers. Moreover, sometimes caregivers found themselves in situations in which emergency medical personnel did not know how to respond. A mother who called an ambulance when her ventilator-dependent son felt he could not breathe said, "*That's* where the anxiety—the frustration comes in. Because the paramedics come and go, 'What am I supposed to do?'" In these situations, caregivers may find themselves taking lead roles in medical assistance, even in the presence of medical personnel. As Phoebe described it, "I was being doctor, nurse, judge, everything."

Notwithstanding situations such as these, which added additional stressors, in general, the caregivers in this book said they did speak up and demand quality care when dealing with medical professionals. Many were tenacious in advocating for their loved ones. For example, several said they had left doctors, or spoken up to home health agencies about nurses, if they did not display what they considered to be caring attitudes. This caregiver explained how she took action when she did not feel that a home health nurse was giving proper care: "She was rough and mean. . . . So we called and complained and told 'em never to send her back again. . . . They did not send her back anymore after that."

Although the pattern among the caregivers in this book was that they displayed such agency, it is important to remember that others may not feel that they have the knowledge or authority to question medical professionals. There is still much more need for research, particularly regarding members of marginalized groups, such as racial and ethnic minorities, and those of varying sexual orientations and gender identities, who may feel they lack the power to make their voices heard (see, for example, Malat and Hamilton 2006). Moreover, clearly, the U.S. health care structure places this care on families, and complaints about individuals or issues go only so far in resolving systematic shortcomings. Due to these factors, as well as the fact that caregivers may feel they have varying abilities to display agency, it is especially important to examine nurses' perceptions and identities in the labor transfer. The ways in which nurses frame their labor have enormous consequences for their interactions with all caregivers. In the next section I explore these dynamics by drawing on existing literature and probing the perspectives of home health nurses.

Nurses' Emotional Labor and Professional Identity

In studying the identity and emotional labor of nurses, it is important to note that the nursing profession itself has wrestled with issues of professionalization—which is often seen as being in the shadows of the professionalization of medical doctors (Porter 1992a; ten Hoeve, Jansen, and Roodbol 2013).[3] Moreover, the definition of nursing as both a "scientific process" and an "art dedicated to caring" (NCSBN 2011b, 3) has been greatly scrutinized. Prior scholarship has held that caring is at the core of nursing's professional identity, and "sentimental" work (Strauss et al. 1982) is often noted as an important component of nursing practice. Yet scholars have also argued that the nursing profession has prioritized caring rhetoric, or what Gordon and Nelson call the "virtue script," to the detriment of understanding the knowledge and complex cognitive work and emotional skills that are required to be a nurse (Gordon 2006; Gordon and Nelson 2006). Gordon (2006, 119) makes the point that nurses' relationships with patients are formed based on the intimate knowledge a nurse amasses through applying highly technical skills to the human body. Theodosius (2008, 33) argues that the physical care that nurses are required to provide makes their emotional labor distinctly different from that of other service workers, and that a "collaborative and therapeutic relationship" between nurses and patients or their relatives may involve "care needs" that are "both complex and long term."

In understanding nurses' identity and their orientation to the work transfer, it is thus important to understand these intricate work processes—processes that are both highly cognitive and emotional. It is true that the nurses I interviewed often talked about their own identities as rooted in caring as being a primary reason for entering the profession: "That's why I'm a nurse—it's just the caring part of it." "I like to help people. . . . It's my passion. It's what God has designed me to do." Indeed, care work scholars note that both paid and unpaid care workers may experience such intrinsic forms of motivation, such as for those who have a "calling that represents a source of deep personal meaning" (England, Folbre, and Leana 2012, 24). Recognizing such motivation, however, should never minimize the complexity and difficulty of the work that must be done. As noted throughout this book, nurses perform complex forms of both cognitive and emotional labor (see Gordon 2006; Gordon and Nelson 2006) in the transfer of their skills.

In understanding the power dynamics in interactions with family caregivers, a major question is how nurses can so freely transfer the knowledge they have taken so long to acquire. How do they feel about turning over their labor to lay caregivers? Are they giving something away? Are they participating in the de-skilling of their own profession? How is the transfer related to their professional identities?

These questions have received little research attention since Glazer (1993) first described the "work transfer" of skilled nursing to family caregivers. She focused on the cost savings realized by capitalist and state organizations as (mostly) unpaid women assumed the work once provided by paid professionals, and she suggested that this process would contribute to nurses' deprofessionalization. In 2003, in one of the few empirical studies of this transfer, Ward-Griffin and Marshall studied twenty-three Canadian female caregivers of the frail elderly and their home health nurses. They found that nurses were able to gradually transfer the skilled labor through strategies such as "gently encouraging" or "forcefully 'pushing' " caregivers to learn, and "if the caring work appeared too difficult or technical, nurses simplified or 'downplayed' these aspects, or they would insist that the caregiver was 'smart enough' to learn" (2003, 199). The authors argued that nurses were "ideological workers" who influenced caregivers through "covert forms of power" that regarded caring as naturally female and part of family obligations (201). They cautioned that their study was socialist-feminist in nature, and had limitations in that it emphasized oppression (in this case of caregivers) without considering individual agency or resistance strategies (204).

A central question of this book is whether, as workers who are embedded in social structure, nurses are "ideological workers," as Ward-Griffin and Marshall suggest—workers who covertly enact power and draw on gender ideologies in transferring their skills. It is certainly true that structural factors and cultural and gender ideologies shape the expectations and actions of both nurses and caregivers—as they do all of us—in ways that structure home and work lives.[4] It is also true that gender is embedded in organizations such as hospitals and the medical establishment (Acker 1990). Yet overly structural views obscure the dynamics of relationships, and the agency, emotional labor, and identities of actors. These concepts are critical in understanding work processes and how skilled labor is transferred (see Hochschild 2003; Burawoy 1979).

Notably, the nurses I interviewed for this book did not generally evoke gender ideologies as a rationale for the transfer of their labor. Several stated that they teach a considerable number of men how to do skilled nursing and that often men do a "fine job." Les said, "I've seen elderly men taking care of their bedbound, stroke wife . . . forever. I've seen younger men do the IVs for their wife." Many nurses, however, understood that caregiving falls disproportionately on women, and they often referred to caregivers as "she," reflecting both their experience and the more likely scenario. Nurses also did not generally downplay the complexity of the labor. In speaking about possible complications from giving IVs, a nurse told me, "They could forget to prime their tubing. . . . You forget to do things when you're nervous and it's your first couple of times. You could kill somebody with an air embolism."[5]

In describing communication with caregivers, nurses often stated that the goal was to make patients and families "independent" in their care. While the cultural construct of "independence" is entangled in gender ideology because independence requires unspoken work, it was the reality of payer sources (no doubt produced by such ideology) that most structured labor processes. Nurses understood the business side of care: "We document for dollars." "We couldn't stay in business if we went out every day." However, they were often at odds with these structural limitations. They were frustrated when payer sources limited their time to teach. In referring to the time limits placed on caregivers who administer IVs, one nurse commented, "I don't think they should . . . have a set amount of time. If it takes six times, then it takes six times. If the nurse has to administer all of them—they have to."

The structural limitations for both caregivers and nurses are critical in understanding the skilled labor transfer. Indeed, in a 2006 study in Ontario, Canada, Oudshoorn, Ward-Griffin, and McWilliam analyzed the power dynamics in four triads—each consisting of a nurse, a family member, and a care recipient—who were involved in home palliative services. Following Giddens (1977, 1984), they found that nurses, family members, and care recipients were all caught in a "hierarchy of power" in which nurses, as well as caregivers, experienced both power and powerlessness (Oudshoorn, Ward-Griffin, and McWilliam 2007, 1438). This analysis is germane to the situation I find with nurse/caregiver/care recipient interactions. All are working within a social structure in which health and social policies dictate many of the resources.

In fact, because nurses realize that structural policies set limits on their labor, they use this knowledge to advocate for patients—for example, by doing as much teaching as they can early on, "front loading" their labor (see chapter 2). In teaching the labor, nurses are also likely to engage in communication that has the effect of reducing their own status in order to show caregivers that the labor can be learned. They said they did not want to come in and "talk above their heads." They sought common ground, and a common language, and gave emotional encouragement and praise when procedures were performed correctly (see chapter 2).

Many nurses expressed great empathy for caregivers who, due largely to insurance limits, had to learn procedures quickly. A nurse told me, "I've seen them in tears, or 'What am I going to do? I can't do this on my own. I'm trying the best I can, I just don't understand it.'" In this situation the nurse tries to encourage the caregiver and "build them up": "'I know this is difficult and I know you're scared to do it. But if we sit down and we talk about it and I write everything down for you, and I watch you a couple of times, I know that you can do this.'"

The emotional encouragement by nurses is especially interesting in light of Theodosius's (2008) work. She finds that although nurses have power over patients, their own emotional labor and professional ideals of good care counterbalance this power. (See Erickson and Stacey [2013] for a discussion.) According to Theodosius (2008, 33–34), the public trusts nurses to be genuinely concerned about health and well-being, and this allows patients to trust that nurses (as strangers) will provide good care.

Furthermore, although nurses are in a position of power over caregivers in regard to their knowledge, as we have seen, caregivers may also display agency—for example, in voicing concerns about nurses to their employers.[6] These findings exemplify what care work scholars have noted as the current context in which care workers practice emotional labor—contexts in which both care and commerce are "operating simultaneously" (Erickson and Stacey 2013, 180).

As stated, the nature of nurses' emotional labor is important in that it speaks to nurses' orientation toward their interactions with caregivers as well as the importance of identity work in the skills transfer. Importantly, the nurses in this book described engaging in all of Bolton and Boyd's (2003) types of emotional labor (see chapter 5). When they discussed their respect of homes and the importance of arriving on time, they said, "We're the guests," and families "don't want you to be the cable man . . . waiting all day for this wound care" (presentational emotional labor). They referred to the importance of maintaining good relationships so the customer is satisfied, or so they "don't get any bad feedback" (pecuniary emotional labor—although this form of emotional labor was seldom discussed). Nurses described caregivers and care recipients becoming "almost like family"—which a nurse called "one of the best, best feelings," when she went on her own time and sat with a daughter whose father was dying because "I had grown close to them and they had grown close to me, and they felt comfortable and secure with me there" (philanthropic emotional labor, or "the gift"). Overall, it was the prioritization of quality patient care as essential to the nurses' identity and to their fulfillment of professional occupational rules (prescriptive emotional labor) that was most salient. "I realize who I'm employed for," one nurse said. "But the reason I'm employed . . . is because of these patients. If it wasn't for the patient, I wouldn't be employed, period. . . . My main goal as a nurse is to come in and take care of the patient."

As this quote demonstrates, nurses—like caregivers—focus foremost on the health and well-being of care recipients. Thus, just as caregivers judge nurses whom they deem not caring, nurses also judge caregivers based on this standard (see chapter 2). A nurse told me that if a family member seems distracted or tries to do errands while she is there, she tells him or her, "This ain't happening."

The prioritization of care recipient health was also used in framing nurses' viewpoints about caregiver independence. Although nurses were critical when patients were sent home "too soon" or without proper instruction, they expressed their belief that, if it is at all possible for care recipients to be at home, they are better off and have better outcomes there: they are "less anxious," have "more freedom," can "get more rest," and can "heal better." Although cleanliness can be an issue in home care (see chapter 4), nurses also said that patients are safer at home because "you don't have all those germs floating around"—particularly "superbugs" or hospital-acquired bacteria. Said Les, "We don't like to send patients to the hospital. We want 'em . . . in good shape. Sometimes they come back with infections, and it's [because] they're around so many other patients."

Nurses also pointed out the advantages of home care for care recipients' emotional health. They compared home care to the hospital, where "you have a different nurse every day." According to Rachel, in home care "you can focus all your attention on that problem, that person." Karen said, "It's not like on the floor where you have eight patients, one nurse, call lights going off constantly. I know when I have that one patient, they have my undivided attention and so does their family. Their emotional needs get met."

Nurses thus draw heavily on the ability of home care to provide holistic nursing practices.[7] According to Les, "You can see the whole person . . . the whole picture, the whole . . . psychosocial atmosphere of the patient."[8] Nurses value home care for its ability to provide unstructured time in the patient's environment, which they believe allows them to better understand patient health and compliance (see also Marrone 2003; Cain 2015). Referring to doctors, hospitals, and insurance companies, one nurse commented, "They don't see what we see at home." Karen said,

> You don't know that they don't have running water. You don't know they don't have a car. You don't know that they can't get to the doctor. You don't know that they don't have food in their cabinets. . . . It's the holistic view that influences their overall health, or I feel that it does, and I think most nursing theorists agree. . . . You don't know why a diabetic has trouble until you see their fixed income and their education level. They don't buy the right foods because they go to the food bank every month and that's just not the foods that are available to them. . . . There's a lot of different things that go on, and until you get to know the family, you don't understand that.

Nurses' focus on patients' physical and emotional health refutes a vision of nurses as purely "ideological workers"—an image that implies an insensitive and coercive nature in the transfer of skills. My analysis of both structural and interactional components confirms the conclusion that both the nurses and the caregivers I studied are interacting within a power structure, in which both prioritize the needs of care recipients.

Moreover, examining both macro- and microcomponents within the unique context of home care (key elements in Erickson and Stacey's [2013] emotion practice theory) sheds light on the transfer of skills. In this regard, nurses contrasted the work processes in home care with those in institutions.[9] Unlike in a hospital, in home care, the relationship between nurses and caregivers is structured by the assumption that caregivers will take over the labor, and nurses recognize the pivotal role of the family caregiver in achieving their highest immediate professional goal—gaining care recipient independence. Thus, rather than experiencing reluctance in relinquishing their skills, they see the transfer as an important element of their professional responsibility. According to Olivia, "On a day-to-day basis . . . we depend on family often to provide the care." As Mildred says, "You couldn't do your job without them."

This interactive and relational component of the work process belies the notion that nurses are merely conduits of professional knowledge. Indeed, because of the integral role of family caregivers, who interact daily with care recipients, nurses told me that it is important to listen to them. If something is wrong, "they would know," a nurse said. Some nurses also said that if caregivers have found efficient or effective ways of implementing procedures at home, they share that knowledge with other families. A home health nurse who visited a caregiver who was caring for a child with complex medical issues told me, "The mom is wonderful. I tell any new nurse, 'If you don't know, ask Mom.'" Thus, while expertise and skilled labor is, without a doubt, transferred from paid professionals to lay caregivers, a unilateral or top-down method of transferring the labor does not fully describe the ways in which labor and teaching processes unfold across private and public domains.[10]

The relationship between nurses and caregivers is indeed critical for nurses, who identify heavily with the education component of their profession. They view themselves as teachers who share a common goal of helping the caregiver learn so that the care recipient can heal. Cecile told me, "I love sitting down with patients and teaching, I just love doing that, you know?" And Tara said, "I like to teach. I've thought about being a clinical instructor . . . for nursing students. I just can't fit it in right now." Because nurses see their role as to evaluate, assess, and teach, instructing lay caregivers does not seem to make them feel "deprofessionalized"—on the contrary, they appear to gain satisfaction from seeing caregivers learn. When discussing what she liked about her job, a nurse said, "I like the relationships I get with all the families and especially if you get them to the point where they don't need you anymore—that's always good."

The Organization of Work and "Surplus Care"

The explication of caregiver and nurse interactions and identities illuminates the mechanisms at play in the skilled care transfer. As shown, interactions occur within an existing social structure, with both caregivers and nurses focusing on care recipient health, and home health nurses identifying with the educational component of their labor.

The study of these interactions between paid professional nurses and largely unpaid lay caregivers is an important addition to prior work on home care aides (Stacey 2005, 2011). Stacey (2011, 102) observes how home care aides are in the contradictory position of being paid workers who are also "fictive kin."[11] She found that home care aides experienced autonomy and found dignity (Hodson 2001) and deep meaning in their jobs, but also experienced " 'losing themselves' " or "overinvesting in client care" (Stacey 2011, 66). They experienced emotional labor negatively when treated as "glorified maids," or when they performed extra work—what Stacey calls "surplus care"—"being asked to stay a little longer for dinner, lend a little money, or take on a little more cooking and cleaning beyond the terms of their contract" (79).

The occupational status of home health nurses sets them apart from home care aides who do not enjoy the same resources. There are some similarities, however. Much like Stacey's aides, the home care nurses I interviewed said they enjoy a great deal of job autonomy and flexibility.[12] Increased autonomy led to positive elements of identity. In order to do home health care, they said, a nurse must be "independent," must be "competent in . . . skills . . . judgment . . . [and] critical thinking," and must have extensive prior experience. Some described home health nurses as having a "unique personality" or as being a "special breed," because they are able to work unsupervised. As one nurse said, "You've gotta be prepared to make something out of nothing." This sense of control may help to reduce negative aspects of emotional labor and job stress (see Wharton 1993).[13]

Also, like Stacey's aides, nurses frequently walk a fine line in dealing with family dynamics, and they are sometimes asked to give surplus care such as taking vital signs for family members who are not the patient. However, nurses have the advantages of professional occupational feeling rules and resources that help them to define their labor and to set boundaries. For example, a nurse told me that if a family member who is not a patient asks her to take his or her vital signs, she replies that she will do so one time, but after that, this care is not within the scope of her services. Occupational status also helps nurses manage their emotional labor. For example, several said they are able to refer families to social workers if they need additional resources or if there are emotional issues. Nurses are also able to cope with the emotional aspects of their jobs by relying on colleagues to discuss their emotions and to vent. Cecile told me, "I . . . talk to other colleagues . . . that sharing of 'What would you do if this?' Or, 'I'm having this kind of problem.' " Korczynski (2003) has called this collective behavior "communities of coping" (see also Lewis 2005; McGuire 2007; Leppänen 2008).

An important component of the skilled labor process, however, is that despite being able to draw on organizational and professional rules and resources, the nurses I interviewed do give surplus care. These cases involve work that is in relation to care recipient health. According to Rose, if a care recipient has not been doing well, and he or she is in the vicinity of a nurse's daily route, "It's not uncommon for your nurse to walk in your door . . . to see if your antibiotic's helping. . . . A lot of people in home health volunteer time."

Indeed, many nurses said they "go over" on their "own time" or "eat the cost" if they feel someone needs help. Nurses discussed calling families after hours to "make sure they're doing okay," giving out cell phone numbers so families will not have to deal with bureaucratic channels, and visiting patients in the hospital, although this was not a requirement of their agencies. Ruth filled medicine planners on her own time for a patient who didn't have a caregiver.[14]

Further, the nature of this surplus care often includes "support care," which, although related to health, would not be considered "skilled nursing." Several nurses said they have taken prescriptions to the pharmacy, picked up medicines or groceries, or fixed light meals when the care recipient was hungry and needed help. One nurse "arranged a lady's furniture . . . to make things a little bit safer," another "threw in laundry," and still another took "tap water in milk jugs" to a home "so they would have some clean water."

Nurses also buy supplies with their own money. One "bought a pillbox" and once "gave a lady who had no insurance" money to buy her pills. Others spend money on cleaning supplies in order to wash down areas and create clean spaces. A nurse administrator told me that even though nurses in her agency are not supposed to buy supplies with their own money, she often finds out that they do, and she compared this process to teachers who buy classroom supplies with their own funds.

When nurses "volunteer" time, money, and resources, they are attempting to meet needs they observe that are not recognized by the system. They give this surplus care in response to needs they deem legitimate, in order to keep patients safe and well. Nurses did not discuss this labor in ways that indicated a negative impact on their identities, but were able to define it as part of their overall professional occupational identity of ensuring patient health and safety—even though they were much outside their job descriptions. Recognizing nurse actions in filling system gaps is crucial in understanding the variability in home life and the issues in providing skilled care there.

Final Thoughts on Emotion Work, Identity, and the Structure of Health Care

Both caregivers and nurses practice complex forms of emotional labor as an intricate part of the multifaceted and often difficult medical procedures they enact. Yet both are working in a system that often constrains their choices. The transfer of the labor, however, is not just structural, but interactive and relational. It has to do with the identities of caregivers who come into the labor process because of their relationships, and nurses who prioritize patient care as part of their professional identities and embrace a role of teacher/educator. It is the related emotion work of caregivers, as well as the emotional labor of paid nurses, that helps facilitate the transfer of skilled labor from the public to the private domain.

Importantly, my interview data reveal that both caregivers and nurses prioritize the well-being of care recipients. This is why caregivers push themselves and why nurses give surplus care. It is for this reason that caregivers demand good care, and nurses respect caregivers who they believe truly care for the care recipient. Indeed, it is the care recipient to whom the actions and emotion work of both caregivers and nurses are directed, and this care process—albeit in different ways—is a central part of identity for each.

Once when I, alongside a registered nurse, was drawing up IV medication at my dining room table, I had a realization: "We are doing the same work." In these last two chapters I have tried to explore more fully the meaning of work for caregivers and nurses.

Although caregivers derive positive impacts on their selfhood, they are still performing hard and demanding work. In the "public" workplace, "job satisfaction" and experiences that positively influence identity are not taken as discounts of the work; if anything, they are desired features of jobs. Indeed, many of the nurses I spoke with enjoy positive professional identities from enacting, and especially teaching, this complex labor to others.

Yet the context of home as a venue for a shared labor process—a process that takes place between paid and unpaid workers (Glazer 1990, 1993)—provides challenges and undeniable gaps in resources, gaps that nurses strive to fill. Understanding the physical and emotional complexities of the skilled care labor process is paramount in deriving policies that incorporate—as Lopez (2006) found in institutions—organized emotional care in which all workers have time to recognize and value the emotional components of this complex labor. Such policies will benefit caregivers and care recipients alike.

Conclusion

It is ironic that I began this study with a description of a flowing meadow. Since then, I have learned that critics often use the image of "silos" to describe the current patchwork system of health care in the United States. Indeed, the system is not a free-flowing, seamless delivery of care between the farmhouse, the hospital, and the payer sources that govern the work performed, but a series of stand-alone silos disbursed across the landscape—some quite distant and others out of view entirely. To find and enter these spaces, you have to negotiate a difficult journey without the help of a map, much less a field guide. In the numerous pathways between the house and the hospital, a world at the intersection of public and private domains, caregivers become active agents who problem solve, devise new work strategies, and fight for resources. They learn and execute work that many home care aides are not legally allowed to perform and that some medical personnel have not been trained to do. Yet society has paid little attention to the labor processes they enact.

As feminist scholars have noted,[1] in the intersections of paid and unpaid worlds, demarcations between public and private seem blurred and false, and caregivers of various backgrounds, abilities, resources, and races and ethnicities find themselves here. Patterns of gender are evident. The addition of skilled caregiving may solidify preexisting patterns of work, or challenge them as families look honestly at who can perform the care work, and what resources are available. While men perform skilled care, and face many of the same challenges as women, one striking pattern is the multiplicity of the caregiving roles of women—they are often caregivers for children, for care recipients with chronic illnesses or disabilities, and for the elderly. They are also generally more loosely tied to the labor market and are more often threatened at their workplaces. Women are also more likely the helpers and advisers of care in the public/private intersection (see chapter 4).

Notably, caregivers' journeys with care recipients reflect varied experiences in interactions with medical professionals and in the training they receive. While some receive excellent training prior to discharge, others receive very little—a pattern that home health nurses observe all too often. Home health nurses see cases where discharge instructions have clearly not been explicitly communicated, and where people are even unaware of the work they must perform at home. Training can significantly impact caregiver confidence and expectations, and an important part of home health nurses' labor is to manage expectations and assess whether caregivers are really "willing and able" to perform the care.[2]

The caregivers I talked with were very concerned that procedures were performed correctly. With little professional oversight, they had to determine whether they were competent to do this new and often frightening work and that they did not negatively impact the health of a loved one. Hiring help could be problematic, not only because of the cost, but also because technically the procedures require a "skilled" nurse, and others may be afraid to take on the tasks. Moreover, homes are not standard—in their resources, their relationships, their family dynamics, or their cleanliness and organization. Caregivers are not the same—in their anxiety, their orientation to the labor, their past experiences, their relationships with care recipients, the social support they receive, their power in the home, or their propensity toward nursing. Attempting to apply standardized measures and allowances of only so many home health visits is problematic in its conception as well as in its application.[3]

With so many variables, how is it that skilled home care is accomplished as often as it is? Though many caregivers experience feelings of anxiety and worry, they say they "do what they have to do" to provide care for those they love. Thus, it is the relationship with the care recipient that motivates their labor, and despite some ambivalent feelings, many have strong feelings against institutionalization. The eyes of caregivers in this study were pointed squarely toward the care recipients, on whom they bestowed dignity and the hope of a meaningful, and to the best of their ability normal, life.

Nurses, through their care work and the application of professional ethics and identity, also say their primary focus is on the welfare of care recipients. They believe home care enhances patient care because they can see patients in a holistic manner. They say they enjoy the autonomy of their jobs and have satisfaction in seeing care recipients and families maintain independence. Although they recognize the needs of caregivers and often provide surplus care, make recommendations, or try to obtain social services, there are times when they face dilemmas and feel bad when their visits to teach or to perform care are limited by payer sources. Moreover, although caregiver experiences with home health nurses vary—from caregivers depending greatly on nurses to caregivers critiquing nurses as being in a hurry, or as unable to educate them on the medical condition of care recipients—both caregivers and nurses seem to evaluate each other based on their perceived care for the care recipient. Examining the emotional labor and identities of caregivers and nurses allows us to see that skilled home health labor processes are accomplished because caregivers—as well as nurses—focus primarily on care recipients' welfare.

Importantly, the caregivers I interviewed had been successful at performing skilled nursing labor. The changing role of home health and the current medical system leaves few alternatives, other than hospitalization or institutionalization. However, although interviews with nurses show that most people do learn the skills, clearly there are cases where there is great reluctance, where people do not feel they have the ability to learn, and where family members do not wish to perform this kind of care for people they love. Moreover, there are people who are not in the best of relationships. There are also situations of abuse or neglect in the home and varying family dynamics, which may make home care a less than ideal situation for caregivers and care recipients alike. Pushing medical procedures home is not always feasible, and people shouldn't be made to feel bad when they can't do it, don't feel that it is right to do it, or quite frankly are afraid to do it. A nurse I spoke with made this point explicitly when she told me she often encourages the medical residents in her hospital to think critically about the almost automatic push toward home care. As she said, "Can I put a tube down my own kid's nose? Every day if I need to? I don't know if I can do that or not."

Moreover, it is not simply a matter of learning skills but of maintaining the necessary tasks over time. Home life itself is dynamic, and caregivers must integrate care with their daily lives. Depending on the length and timing of care, caregivers may spend considerable amounts of time giving care. They may also suffer economic hardship, job loss, anxiety, and constraints in exploring other avenues of positive identity development. In a society that has largely tied benefits to paid work, we are not making way for the reality of caregiving experiences in the lives of women or men.

We need to make better accommodations and recognize the inevitability of sickness, accidents, and death as part of the human experience (Kittay 1999). Currently the U.S. has individualized solutions to care and provides very few comprehensive welfare solutions for families (Meyer, Herd, and Michel 2000). Moreover, as Meyer, Herd, and Michel (2000, 3) maintain, making individual families responsible for care exacerbates socioeconomic inequalities. Kittay (1999, 12–13), in building a philosophical framework for caring, discusses the feminist "diversity critique," which calls attention to the intersection of race, gender, class, age, and disability in examining inequality, and recognizes that not all men are equal to each other, just as not all women are equal to each other (see hooks 1987). As a critical response to this critique, Kittay (1999, 13–14) offers the "dependency critique," which also recognizes that we cannot discuss individual rights without realizing that the "human condition" and the formation of deep relationships—which define our humanity—create asymmetry.[4] According to Kittay, while we are familiar with ideals of "individual-based equality," we need to move to a stance that recognizes and strives for "connection-based equality," which recognizes interdependency and takes into account the inevitability of our caring relationships with others (28). As she points out, we need to realize that someone must take care of those who need it, and "we need to ask whether doing dependency work excludes those who do it from the class of equals, and if so, what we must understand and do to end this exclusion" (16). Likewise, Duffy, Stacey, and Armenia (2015, 291) contend that care should be regarded as "a critical part of human infrastructure and as a basic ethical obligation of society." Doing so, they maintain, will transform "this ethic of care from an individual responsibility to a collective imperative."

So how can we effect positive change for families who are enacting skilled medical labor and improve the work process for caregivers, care recipients, and nurses alike? Certainly, robust national policies that support family care work are in order. To begin, we should ensure transparent, dependable, transportable, and understandable quality health care coverage, including home health benefits, for all Americans. Not only preserving the vital protections in the ACA but also working for better accessibility and lower costs should be a top national priority. Americans should know their benefits and not have to navigate the current maze of payer sources and waiver systems. Citing the current complexity of U.S. public care policy, including the "perverse incentives to shift costs between federal, state, and local programs," Folbre, Howes, and Leana (2012, 185–86) argue for "relatively universal care policies, where taxpayers can clearly see what they are getting for their money." Indeed, we need to move toward health policies that cover all Americans and are not stratified by socioeconomic and demographic variables or the nuances of state insurance mandates.

Caregivers also need consistent and standard training, and they need to understand what they will be up against at home. In April 2019, the AARP Public Policy Institute released *Home Alone Revisited*, an update to its 2012 *Home Alone* survey.[5] The 2019 report summarized major findings from a national online survey of 2,089 caregivers, about half of whom performed medical/nursing tasks (Reinhard, Young, Levine, et al. 2019). The results corroborate many of the findings and conclusions in this book. Caregivers who were performing nursing tasks wanted better instruction, and more than half were performing three or more tasks. The greater the complexity of the tasks, the more caregivers worried about making mistakes (34). Sleep disturbances were reported by about six in ten caregivers (23). Women were more likely than men to feel stressed because of multiple responsibilities, including caring for other family members or work commitments (25). Other findings included the identification of pain management as a major issue that created emotional strain (36), and the importance of understanding the diversity of caregivers in terms of age and sociocultural demographics. For example, millennials were twice as likely as baby boomers to note that tasks were difficult to perform (19), and members of nonwhite racial and ethnic groups were more likely to experience strain and worry about making a mistake, regardless of their income (20).[6] These findings highlight the need for future research into multiple populations and at-risk groups to understand their unique experiences with performing complex care.

Regarding hospital training and communication, the work of the AARP Public Policy Institute, in conjunction with multiple federal and state stakeholders, including caregiver organizations, has led to promising initiatives. AARP drafted model state legislation called the CARE (Caregiver Advise, Record, Enable) Act, which has become law in forty states and territories (Reinhard, Young, Ryan, et al. 2019, 1). Although the state provisions and names of specific acts vary, in general, hospitals in these states must

> *advise* individuals of their opportunity to identify a family caregiver, *record* the caregiver's name and contact information in the health record (with the patient's permission) and *enable* family caregivers by providing as much notice as possible about discharge timing, consulting with them about the discharge plan, discussing their role in carrying out that plan, and instructing them about the medical/nursing tasks they will handle at home. (2)

To better understand implementation of the CARE Act, follow-up site visits were conducted in eighteen health systems and forty-seven hospitals in nine U.S. states. Through discussions with key stakeholders,[7] the visits identified major themes, including the use of electronic health records to identify and include caregivers, innovative strategies such as "team huddles" to broaden communication, staff training on caregiver inclusion, innovative instruction such as videos and teach-back sessions, better discharge coordination including follow-up calls, and the identification of caregivers and populations who may need additional support, such as those with language and cultural considerations or certain medical conditions.[8] In general, the authors found that CARE Act benefits included "greater satisfaction and confidence with care transitions, reduced unnecessary rehospitalizations, and improved quality outcomes" (8). They also noted that future follow-up studies will identify and elevate promising practices.

The CARE Act should be celebrated as a long overdue recognition of the role of caregivers and a move toward better hospital training and discharge processes. There are states, however, in which it still has not been implemented. Moreover, the 2019 *Home Alone Revisited* report, cited above, showed that eight out of ten caregivers received less than twenty-four hours' notice about discharge, and only three out of five reported receiving instruction prior to discharge, with men less likely to receive instruction than women (Reinhard, Young, Levine, et al. 2019, 29–30). Future evaluations are needed to reveal more about CARE Act compliance and effectiveness.

Moreover, an important point is that it is not just a matter of learning the tasks, but of performing them at home and maintaining them over time amid the fragmented national system. We need to ensure adequate, ongoing support at home for all caregivers. Certainly, having credentialed nurses and health care professionals make regular home visits and providing more in-home support are essential. Nurses see the reality of the home situation and face inconsistencies that complicate the provision of care. Their working knowledge should be reintegrated into the health care system to a much greater extent than it currently is. Nurses should be allowed to exercise professional judgment to make the number of visits they deem necessary, and to stay as long as they deem necessary, without the fear of being cut off by insurance caps.

Carol Levine at the United Hospital Fund has been a strong advocate for the idea that nurses, social workers, and other professionals also "need better tools to truly assess, systematically and without stereotypes, each caregiver's strengths and limitations. They need tools to help caregivers find resources and plan for services that will compensate for limitations" (2006, 43). Writing in the *American Journal of Nursing*, Levine makes the point that leaders in social work and nursing need a better educational curriculum, one that takes into account "not only what the care recipient requires, but also what the caregiver is able and willing to provide," as "some caregivers are limited by age, poor health, careers, and other responsibilities and can't do the job alone" (2008, 14–15). Reinhard, Young, Ryan, et al. (2019) advocate for this type of holistic approach in working with caregivers. Although some state caregiver programs have implemented caregiver assessment protocols that consider factors such as self-perceptions of mental health and physical health (Avison et al. 2018),[9] these are not uniform across states, providers, and programs. All caregivers should be able to discuss their own strengths and needs with respect to carrying out the medical work, including factors such as their own employment status and other caregiving roles. Much more needs to be done in order to develop best practices and implementation of standard and meaningful caregiver assessments.[10]

More home support would also increase the confidence of caregivers and reduce emotional burdens. Lessons learned from prior studies of paid work can be applied here. Sociologists and care work and labor scholars have documented how structural and cultural changes within workplaces themselves have a great bearing on the emotional labor and identities of workers (Leidner 1999; Lopez 2006). In his ethnographic study of nursing home aides, Lopez (2006) found that organizations that leave space for employees to truly interact with patients—what he calls "organized emotional care"—produce workplaces in which aides feel fewer emotional burdens from their jobs. Such organizations prioritize giving employees enough time to process work tasks and interact with patients. In this vein, making time for active listening and interaction would be key in addressing some of the structural constraints in home care, where payer source limitations have not allowed adequate time for teaching, learning, and emotional processing. Caregivers need support and time in order to gain confidence and feel assured that they can truly handle the work. Lopez's notion of organized emotional care should be considered in light of the structure of home workplaces in order to promote caregiver and care recipient well-being.

We also need adequate work leave policies for families. The current FMLA offers unpaid family leave if an employee is not able to work due to having a serious health condition or needing to care for a loved one who is seriously ill, or when families have given birth or adopted or fostered a child (USDOL 2019). This leave is limited to twelve weeks and is only for those who work in public agencies, schools, or companies with fifty or more employees, and employees must have worked at least twelve months for at least 1,250 hours in order to qualify (USDOL 2019). There have been many critiques of FMLA. Not only is the leave unpaid, which precludes many families from taking it, but many fall outside the qualifying parameters.[11] Although some states have expanded FMLA through extending time off, reducing the size of workplace requirements, or making definitions of family members more inclusive, and a handful of states provide paid family leave (Gornick, Howes, and Braslow 2012a, 121, 123),[12] the current federal law is simply inadequate and does not capture the real needs of families who are experiencing a health crisis.

Citing the notable lack of federally funded U.S. paid family leave in comparison with peer affluent countries, Folbre, Howes, and Leana (2012) have argued for the development of a national paid family leave program.[13] In 2019, the Family and Medical Insurance Leave (FAMILY) Act was proposed by Rep. Rosa DeLauro (D-CT) and Sen. Kirsten Gillibrand (D-NY). The act would provide caregivers with up to twelve weeks of up to 66 percent of their pay when they take time off due to their own serious illness, childbirth or adoption, or the need to care for a family member with a serious health condition (NPWF 2019, 1). The act would cover full-time, part-time, and self-employed workers, and would be funded through employee and employer payroll contributions of two-tenths of 1 percent each,[14] which is estimated at less than two dollars per week for an average worker (1). Developing a strong federal leave program would acknowledge the reality of care work and demonstrate investment in all citizens.

Much policy work has also documented the inadequacy of long-term care provision in the United States. Many Americans are ill prepared for these expenditures, and they may not realize that they are not covered by Medicare or their insurance, or they are simply unable to afford the insurance premiums for private long-term care coverage (Gornick, Howes, and Braslow 2012b, 149; NHPF 2013, 2). Medicaid, which accounts for about two-thirds of long-term care expenditures (NHPF 2013, 5), generally requires individuals to have limited assets and income, and the application process is complicated and varies greatly by state (NHPF 2013, 2). When Congress, in 2013, tasked the Commission on Long-Term Care (CLTC) to develop a comprehensive long-term care plan, including its financing, the final report recommended actions that we know to be effective in care provision, such as integration of long-term services and supports (LTSS) with other medical services, use of person- and family-centered approaches, standard assessment processes, inclusion of caregivers in care plans, and recognition of the need for support such as training (CLTC 2013; NHPF 2013, 6). The commission, however, could not agree on how to finance long-term care, with some commissioners arguing for market incentives to increase individuals' use of the private market, and others promoting a social insurance approach via the use of Medicare or another public program (NHPF 2013, 7–8). We need to move forward with national policies that recognize long-term care as an issue that many Americans will face, rather than placing burdens on families to research and fund long-term care insurance and continuing our reliance on Medicaid for only those who qualify.

The financial needs of caregivers should also be considered, including their loss of jobs and income. Some states have programs that pay family caregivers for some of their work, and policy scholars have argued for government funding to support family caregivers (Folbre 2012a, xiii; Duffy, Stacey, and Armenia 2015, 289). Medicaid waivers are used by all states to allow those who qualify for self-directed LTSS programs to manage their own care, including hiring caregivers, yet the eligibility and definitions as to what constitutes "caregivers"—including whether or not they can be family members—varies by state, and care recipients must meet income and asset guidelines (AARP 2019). Once again, we are relying on Medicaid programs to select only certain caregivers for specific state programs, stressing the need for national, understandable plans.

Clear, national policies should allow for reasonable compensation and retirement vehicles for those who spend significant time caring for family members. In 2017, Sen. Chris Murphy (D-CT) introduced a proposal to amend Title II of the Social Security Act to give Social Security credit, for up to five years of service, to unpaid caregivers who give care for at least eighty hours per month.[15] This is a much-needed policy; however, a close reading of the bill reveals that a "chronically dependent individual" means a care recipient who needs help with at least two "activities of daily living," such as bathing, or "instrumental activities of daily living," such as meal preparation or help with finances. The need for skilled medical care should be clarified in such legislation; nevertheless, the proposal is a step in the right direction.

Strong national policies should also include caregiver respite. The U.S. falls far behind other countries that have national respite policies (referred to as "short break care") (Rose, Noelker, and Kagan 2015). Rose,

Noelker, and Kagan (2015, 302–3) argue that we should educate caregivers and the public about the need for respite early in the caring career, so as to prevent burnout, adverse health effects, and crises later on. In the U.S., Medicare does not generally provide respite, except for temporary, short-term periods for hospice care (see chapter 3). Other programs for respite vary by state and have experienced reauthorization delays and underfunding from federal sources (305).[16]

The National Family Caregiver Support Program (NFCSP), which is managed through the Administration for Community Living (ACL), gives grants to states for caregiver support, including respite, but these are only for caregivers who meet certain demographic criteria. Funding amounts to states and territories are based on the percentage of the population that is age seventy and older, and are for adults ages eighteen or over who care for family members who are sixty or over, or who have Alzheimer's. Relatives age fifty-five or older who care for children under the age of eighteen (of whom they are not the parents), or for adults (including their own children) ages eighteen to fifty-nine who have disabilities, are also covered (ACL 2019b). The NFCSP has supported vital programs but is drastically underfunded, receiving $145,586,000 in 2013–2015 and $150,586,000 in 2016 (ACL 2019b), far short of the billions of dollars needed (Rose, Noelker, and Kagan 2015, 305). The federal Lifespan Respite Care Act, which was signed into law in December 2006 and is also administered through the ACL, "addresses family caregiver respite issues, regardless of age or disability," but again, the bill has not been well funded and has experienced reauthorization delays (Rose, Noelker, and Kagan 2015, 304–5). Although thirty-seven states and the District of Columbia have received grants, the average appropriation has been only about $2.5 million per year since 2009 (ACL 2019a), with funding of $4.1 million in 2018 and 2019 (ARCH 2019b). The Lifespan Respite Care Reauthorization Act was introduced in April 2019 by Sen. Susan Collins (R-ME) and Sen. Tammy Baldwin (D-WI), and in the House by Rep. Jim Langevin (D-RI) and Rep. Cathy McMorris Rodgers (R-WA), and authorizes $200 million over five years for states to implement coordinated systems of respite care, including training respite workers and providing education to caregivers on how to access services. The bill, however, currently awaits reauthorization (ARCH 2019b).

Such delays, and a lack of funding overall, are especially troubling because programs for respite and training have shown improvement in caregiver outcomes. A 2018 evaluation by the NFCSP program used three telephone surveys conducted in 2016–2017 to compare NFCSP client caregivers and a comparison group who did not use NFCSP services (Avison et al. 2018). Results showed that "caregivers who received 4 or more hours of respite care per week had a decrease in self-reported burden over time, while the comparison caregivers experienced an increase in self-reported burden" (xix).[17] Moreover, NFCSP caregivers "who attended at least one education/training, counseling, or support group session" experienced an increase in self-reported caregiver confidence, while those who did not receive services showed a decrease in their mean confidence scores (xx).

These analyses emphasize the crucial need for systematic caregiver supports. Policy advocates maintain that programs in countries such as Sweden, in which all caregivers receive four hours per week of respite at no charge, plus a carer's allowance, or Japan, in which respite is provided by long-term care insurance, are examples of what national policies can accomplish (Rose, Noelker, and Kagan 2015, 305). There are also model programs within the United States, particularly the Program of Comprehensive Assistance for Family Caregivers, in the U.S. Department of Veterans Affairs (Rose, Noelker, and Kagan 2015, 306; Gordon 2017, 27). Care recipients are eligible for the program if they have had a serious injury such as traumatic brain injury, or psychological trauma, related to active-duty service on or after September 11, 2001, and need personal care services to perform one or more activities of daily living and/ or need supervision or protection due to lasting neurological damage or injury (USVA 2019c). Caregiver services include education and training, compensation, respite for up to thirty days per year, access to health insurance, travel costs when accompanying the care recipient to medical care, and mental health services and counseling (USVA 2019c).[18]

Moreover, the Veteran Directed Care Program, for enrolled veterans who need nursing skills but want to reside at home, uses consumer-directed decision making about what services are needed, and allows for caregiver pay (USVA 2019a). Through the Aid and Attendance (A&A) program, veterans who need assistance may also be eligible for increased pension amounts (USVA 2019b). Gordon (2017) demonstrates that the Veterans Health Administration (VHA) has been an innovator in providing quality, integrated health care with high satisfaction and outcomes that are at or above those of private providers. Yet the VHA has often been maligned by excessive press coverage about long wait times, while the same attention is not given to wait times for private providers (38–44). Moreover, Gordon finds that not only have VHA wait times improved, but the issues have primarily stemmed from lack of adequate funding rather than problems with quality health care delivery (40–41).

In all, the picture that emerges from U.S. policy work is that we know the kinds of things that help, but we have not taken the initiative to prioritize the care work that Americans are doing. Supporting comprehensive caregiver assessments, and providing resources to fill gaps, will take a society-level ideological and policy shift. Clearly in the United States we have focused on the medical outcomes of care recipients almost exclusively.[19] We have generally treated the care recipient as a stand-alone unit in terms of his or her medical needs and outcomes, without taking a holistic view of the daily realities of living and the resources and time that are involved in maintaining health.

In 2017, the Recognize, Assist, Include, Support, and Engage (or RAISE) Family Caregivers Act received broad bipartisan support and was signed by President Trump in January 2018. The law charges the secretary of health and human services, in consultation with an advisory committee made up of representatives from multiple stakeholders,[20] to review best practices and develop a national Family Caregiving Strategy (AARP 2018).[21] The strategy will seek public input and be made publicly available. Although this is a promising development, the act does not authorize any additional funding, and it is yet to be determined whether a coordinated and well-funded policy implementation will result.

Despite an overall lack of funding and policy implementation in general, we should still acknowledge the progress that has been made, such as state adoptions of the CARE Act. Collective activism brings reason for cautious hope. Groups have formed, such as the National Alliance for Caregiving and the National Family Caregivers Association. Following AARP/United Hospital Fund's 2012 national survey, a Home Alone Alliance, dedicated to caregivers who are performing skilled care at home, was created by the AARP Public Policy Institute, the Betty Irene Moore School of Nursing at

UC Davis, the Family Caregiver Alliance, and the United Hospital Fund (Reinhard, Young, Ryan, et al. 2019, 4). The AARP Public Policy Institute has been working with the Alliance and has published three instructional videos (on wound care, mobility, and managing medications) as well as resource guides for caregivers, and has written articles in the *American Journal of Nursing* (5) that give guidance to nurses who provide at-home instruction. Coalitions such as the ARCH National Respite Network and Resource Center, which works for the development and promotion of respite programs, including helping families to locate services, are doing important work (ARCH 2019a). Yet there is still much more work to do in regard to caregivers' rights and responsibilities. Clearly caregivers who feel they have recognition, a voice, and a choice in their labor are better off.[22] In this regard, the Canadian scholar Patricia McKeever (1999) has said there can be a meaningful coalition between nurses and caregivers. Both are part of a system in which policy and payer sources dictate the amount and timing of the work that is done.

Our current policies have been fragmented, state driven, targeted only to certain care recipients and their caregivers, and highly dependent on complicated Medicaid waivers. It is time to recognize and compensate caregivers for the work they do and to make sure that care recipients also have adequate support. After all, adult care recipients may want and need independence from their families and may prefer to have nonfamily caregivers or to live apart from their families of origin. We need to figure out a national place for home care that moves beyond the institution-versus-family-home dichotomy, and there should be a range of choices for caregivers and care recipients alike. In arguing for national comprehensive care policies, Folbre, Howes, and Leana (2012, 186) point out that critics often claim that public care provision will undermine private provision—a concept known as "crowding out." But they maintain that this thesis "poses a less significant threat than shortfalls in care provision that not only hurt our most vulnerable citizens but also penalize those who take responsibility for the care of others." Building on the work that has been done to date, we do have the ability to implement national policies that benefit all of us. It will require fully realizing the human needs that we have in common and prioritizing those needs.

Thanks to help from many dedicated nurses, therapists, and others, by the time we took our son to college, some three hours from home, he had learned to do his daily care, and felt it important to be independent. I was worried. What if he needed IVs? His year was successful. He made many friends and did very well in classes. Sure enough, at the end of the first school year, he had a hospital admission. After the one-week stay, he was to continue the IVs for one week. We wanted home health to come check on him daily since he was living on his own, and our insurance policy had enough visits to allow for this. My son and husband met the home health nurse on a Saturday, and unfortunately she said she had traveled a distance to get there, had kids of her own, and would not be able to come the next day. Our son wanted to be independent, and for him that meant needing services—not just having his parents do all his IVs. After she left, my husband immediately called the agency, talked to the manager, and told him that after the interaction with the first nurse, we did not want her back. The manager was very distressed to hear of our situation and agreed that someone else would come on Monday and would follow up three days a week. The nurse who came was very professional, and later that week, we got a call from the director of nursing, apologizing for the first nurse's behavior.

In relaying this story, I am reminded of what a caregiver once said to me: "It's a matter of standing up for yourself and saying we're not doing it." Although the caregivers in this book displayed such agency, limitations still mean that caregivers, and even care recipients, are performing a great deal of care on their own. In my son's case, although fortunately he had friends and a sister who helped him, his desire to be independent and stay in school meant he performed much of the IV administration by himself—an exhausting schedule for a college student. Why shouldn't nurses be allowed to come and perform some of the care for care recipients and caregivers who are often on call around the clock? Moreover, some caregivers are in better positions than others to stand up. While this book has looked at both male and female caregivers in different relationships and family formations, and includes cases of single adults, it unfortunately is not able to speak systematically about the experiences of those who are racial or ethnic minorities, or those who are in nontraditional families such as gay- and lesbian-headed households. These caregivers no doubt have many more stories to tell. We need to hear from them.

In many ways, my son's story testifies to a truth voiced by the caregivers as well as many of the home health nurses—who may provide extra or surplus care, or face dilemmas when they cannot: the "independence" we tout requires support. This notion calls on society to realize the beauty, the struggles, the love, and the intense work processes that simultaneously take place in the intersection between public and private worlds. Taking a broadened approach helps us to realize our interdependency, and how the work performed here benefits not only care recipients but society as well. Moreover, this work has unparalleled influence on the ability of caregivers and care recipients to enjoy meaningful lives, as well as to find and sustain employment in "public sphere" jobs. Ultimately this view allows us to see, as feminists have argued, that we are all, at some point, recipients of care.

Methodological Appendix

From January 2009 to February 2010, I interviewed twenty-eight care-givers from twenty-five families (six were spouses who were caring for children), twenty-one registered nurses, and seven other interested parties including two social workers, a case worker, a home health agency administrator, a Medicaid administrator, a home care advocate/lobbyist and a caregiver advocate. I also interviewed six adult care recipients who expressed interest in the project and offered to give their viewpoints. Respondents were interviewed in their homes, in their workplaces, or in coffee shops. Their names and identifying information have been changed in order to protect confidentiality. Interviews generally lasted between one and two hours.

I also had dozens of informal conversations with nurses, social workers, and caregivers. I spent a day and a half in the field—one day riding with home health nurses, and another observing patient teaching in a clinic. I kept abreast of current nursing concerns through discussions with professional nurses and reading bulletins from the American Nurses

Association. I also attended an aging conference, a home health care conference, and caregiver functions, including one caregiver support group.

I purposely recruited caregivers who had performed skilled nursing techniques in taking care of their loved ones. In order to assure consistency in analyzing the labor processes for both nurses and caregivers, I relied primarily on the definitions and descriptions of "skilled nursing care" used in federally funded Medicare regulations on home care. Medicare defines skilled nursing care as "a level of care that includes services that can only be performed safely and correctly by a licensed nurse (either a registered nurse or a licensed practical nurse)" (Medicare 2011). Examples of skilled care for the Medicare home health component include "giving IV drugs, certain injections, or tube feedings; changing dressings; and teaching about prescription drugs or diabetes care" (CMS 2010b, 8). It is important to note that although I generally rely on Medicare definitions, the procedures that government agencies consider "skilled" reimbursable procedures may change over time and may vary by state laws. For example, as discussed in chapter 3, in order to control costs, Medicare no longer considers blood draws in the home to be skilled reimbursable procedures, unless they are performed in conjunction with other skilled procedures, and many patients must now go to labs to have blood drawn. I adopt a view that if caregivers are performing procedures such as blood draws (which indeed one caregiver in this study is doing) that would normally be performed by professionals in a hospital or outpatient setting, they are performing "skilled care" even though a home health nurse would not be reimbursed for this procedure unless it was performed in connection with another skilled procedure.

In an online survey conducted by AARP and the United Hospital Fund after my fieldwork, the authors included the following in their definition of difficult medical and nursing tasks: using incontinence equipment/administering enemas, doing wound care and ostomy care, managing medicines including IVs, preparing food for special diets, operating medical equipment (e.g., ventilators, suctioning equipment, and tube feeding equipment), helping with mobility devices such as canes and walkers, using meters/monitors, and operating durable medical equipment such as hospital beds or lifts (Reinhard, Levine, and Samis 2012, 20). The basis for my sample is a bit more restrictive; for example, I did not use complicated meal preparation, helping with mobility devices, or managing oral medicines as criteria for inclusion. But caregivers often talked of other such complex skills, and these are discussed in context. The result is similar to that of Macdonald (2008), who has defined "medically complex care tasks" as those that involve the operation of technological equipment, the use of sophisticated diagnostic skills, exposure to bodily fluids, and/or substantial risk to care recipients.

In order to reach caregivers who had performed a wide range of nursing skills, I determined which types of illnesses or conditions might require nursing labor and then made contact with caregiver groups and associations in order to let them know about the study. I also received a few other referrals from people who were interested in the study. By opening my study to caregivers who had dealt with multiple illnesses or conditions, and bringing in caregivers from numerous sources, I hoped to increase the variability of the labor performed and the conditions under which it was learned and negotiated. My final sample included caregivers caring for persons with cancer, ALS, cystic fibrosis, spinal cord injury, brain injury, amputation due to diabetes, cerebral palsy, and short bowel syndrome.

Besides varying the particular care work performed, I also allowed the relationship between the caregiver and the care recipient to vary. Of the twenty-eight caregivers, nineteen were parents or guardians, six were spouses, one was a daughter, one a sister, and one an uncle. All caregivers resided with care recipients at the time the care was given. Twenty-two of the caregivers were female and six were male. Their age ranges were thirty-six to forty-five years (n = 6), forty-six to fifty-five years (n = 14), fifty-six to sixty-five years (n = 5), and sixty-six and over (n = 3). Of the twenty-eight caregivers, twenty-four reported education beyond high school as follows: some college (n = 8), technical or associate's degree (n = 7), bachelor's degree (n = 5), and post-bachelor's degree (n = 4). Nine caregivers resided in suburbs and large cities, ten resided in small cities, and nine resided in rural areas. At the time of the interview, seventeen caregivers were married, one was single, and ten were divorced, widowed, or separated. Thirteen had children under the age of eighteen at home. The twenty-eight caregivers resided in twenty-five households with approximate income as follows: less than $25,000 (n = 4), $25,000 to $40,000 (n = 3), $40,000 to $60,000 (n = 6), $60,000 to $100,000 (n = 4), and over $100,000 (n = 8). The majority of the caregivers identified as being white. One caregiver identified as being both white and Native American and one identified as being Asian American. The years spent in caregiving at the time of the interview were as follows: less than one year (n = 4), one to three years (n = 3), three to four years (n = 7), and greater than four years (n = 14).

Research performed in institutional settings has shown that bureaucratic accounts of hospitalizations or procedures often do not tell the full story of interactions and the social processes experienced by patients or their caregivers (see, for example, Diamond 1992). An important strength of this book is its quest to understand caregivers' own versions of their knowledge, competencies, and experiences. Because caregivers were not recruited in conjunction with specific hospital stays or encounters with the medical establishment, they were encouraged to talk broadly about their experiences with multiple care providers in their everyday lives. Therefore, caregivers' quotes reflect their understanding of the processes they enact. The book is not meant to judge the appropriateness or accuracy of the procedures they perform. Moreover, because it focuses on labor processes as a part of the caregiving experience, it does not attempt to analyze health outcomes for care recipients.

I recruited registered nurses in order to better understand the teaching process and home care experience from the paid providers' viewpoint. I located interviewees through initial contacts with nurses who practiced in home health care, and made additional contacts by networking within the nursing profession. Some nurses referred others, and so there were elements of snowball sampling in the process. Of the twenty-one nurses, twenty were female and one was male. Their age ranges were twenty-four years or less (n = 1), twenty-five to thirty-five years (n = 4), thirty-six to forty-five years (n = 5), forty-six to fifty-five years (n = 4), fifty-six to sixty-five years (n = 5), and sixty-six and over (n = 2). All nurses were registered nurses (RNs). Their educational attainment was as follows: technical or associate's degree (n = 11), bachelor's degree (n = 3), and post-bachelor's degree (n = 7). One nurse who had an associate's degree was enrolled in a bachelor's program. Three nurses resided in suburbs and large cities, five resided in small cities, and thirteen resided in rural areas. The place of residence, however, was not necessarily the place of practice. For example, at least two nurses who lived in rural areas at the time of the interview worked part time for home health agencies in large metropolitan areas. At least one nurse who resided in a small city had prior experience in large metropolitan areas. Nurses were encouraged to speak broadly about their experiences, and multiple geographic locations are represented in their accounts. About an equal number of nurses had experience in for-profit and not-for-profit home health agencies. Nurses also had experience in hospitals, community health organizations, and nursing homes. Two had worked as independent providers. At the time of the interview, fourteen of the nurses were married, one was single, and six were divorced, widowed, or separated. Twelve had children under the age of eighteen at home. The twenty-one nurses resided in twenty-one households with approximate income as follows: $25,000 to $40,000 (n = 1), $40,000 to $60,000 (n = 6), $60,000 to $100,000 (n = 5), and over $100,000 (n = 9). All twenty-one nurses identified as being white. Funding allowed for twenty-five-dollar gift cards in consideration of nurses' and caregivers' time.

Nurses provided invaluable triangulation in the research process, and I was able to compare and contrast experiences and perspectives of caregivers with those of nurses throughout the data collection phase. Besides giving insight into teaching methods, nurses also answered questions about the nature of skilled nursing procedures, third-party payer issues, and the home care environment in general. Corroboration by social workers, caseworkers, and administrators was also helpful in this regard.

Despite the study's strengths, it has important limitations. First, my sample is limited to only those caregivers who have actually *performed* skilled nursing labor. No doubt there are countless cases where caregivers do not or cannot perform such labor, and their viewpoints are an important part of the home health debate. While I am not privy to their stories firsthand, in my interviews with nurses they told me about some of the dynamics they have observed. Another important point is that my sample is not representative of the population of caregivers in the United States. In my quest for caregivers who have performed skilled work, I have no doubt captured the experiences of caregivers who have performed more skilled nursing than is demographically true of a "typical" caregiver. Skilled nursing labor is admittedly only one aspect of care work, and many caregivers perform other important work, such as Alzheimer's care, grocery shopping, running errands, advocacy work, and making meals for their elderly or ill family members.

Even more importantly, my sample is not representative of all caregivers in terms of demographic characteristics. For example, while it is true that most of this book's caregivers are middle-aged women—which would be predicted based on demographic data on caregivers at the time of my field work(NAC and AARP 2009, 14–17)—recruiting caregivers through caregiving organizations and referrals may disproportionately capture caregivers who are white and/or of higher socioeconomic status. This has been noted in prior research, and indeed, most caregivers in this book are middle- and upper-middle-class whites. However, the book does offer good cases for comparison with regard to socioeconomic status, and I have been able to illuminate how caregiving affects the ability of caregivers to perform paid work, and how it changes work patterns, particularly for single caregivers. I have also been able to provide a greater understanding of how payer sources stratify and shape labor processes as they directly determine what particular benefits are available to caregivers. Interviews with nurses also shed some light on how caregivers who face educational barriers such as illiteracy are affected in home health processes.

Prior research has documented the salience of race and ethnicity in interactions with the medical establishment. African Americans, for example, are less likely to have access to services and may experience discrimination in interactions with medical providers (Wright and Perry 2010; Malat and Hamilton 2006). Ethnic minorities who have language barriers also face additional obstacles. Further research is definitely needed in order to better understand the experiences of racial and ethnic minorities, and the challenges they face, as they negotiate home health labor, as well as the experiences of those in nontraditional family formations. I hope this book will serve as a springboard in that endeavor.

NOTES

Introduction

1. Smith is referring to the experiences of women within a society that has been dominated and framed by men, and argues that these experiences have not been considered in the development of institutional bases of knowledge.

2. See Tronto's discussion of white women and "the problem of partial privilege" (1993, 17).

3. Feminists have often critiqued the ideological glorification of home and family. According to Thorne (1992, 3, 24), images of middle-class, patriarchal families are often evoked to show that contemporary families are in "crises." Such images, however, obscure the true variations in families, which are due to demographic, economic, and social changes, not moral decline (24). In regard to care work, Abel and Nelson caution that caregiving in the home is "easily romanticized" and that intimate relationships can foster "tensions and conflicts as well as solicitude and warmth" (1990, 8–9).

4. See Folbre (2012b) for a comprehensive discussion of valuation methods and estimates. The AARP places an estimate of $450 billion on unpaid care—and this is only for care that adults (over age eighteen) provide for other adults (Folbre 2012b; Feinberg et al. 2011).

5. The mechanisms of stress are complicated, and studies have used different data sets and measures—sometimes with contradictory findings. For example, one study links caregiving to increased mortality (Schulz and Beach 1999), but another finds that if providing care is measured separately from the stress that is inherent in being exposed to a loved one who has health problems, caregiving activity may actually reduce mortality risk (Brown et al. 2009).

In a review of the literature, Bianchi, Folbre, and Wolf (2012, 59–60) make the case that many stress studies do not consider the positive outcomes of care, suffer from selectivity biases, and lack appropriate comparison groups.

6. See Elmore (2014) for a literature review regarding stresses and benefits.

7. Indeed, home health care has bloomed into a thriving industry. According to a quarterly Bureau of Labor Statistics (BLS) report, "Home healthcare services is projected to be the fastest growing detailed industry in the economy, with employment projected to increase by almost 60 percent between 2012 and 2022" (USDOL 2014, 30). Howes, Leana, and Smith (2012, 82) explore BLS data and find that in terms of employment, home health care and "home care" (services for the elderly and those with disabilities) are the fastest- and second-fastest-growing industries in the U.S.

8. Braverman's work analyzed the plight of paid employees under capitalistic work processes and the Tayloristic control that employers exerted over workplaces.

9. See Graham (1983).

10. Ethnographic research on paid care workers, such as nurses and nurses' aides, has primarily focused on labor processes within institutional settings (Diamond 1992; Foner 1994; Chambliss 1996; Lopez 2004, 2006). Much of this research calls attention to the challenges of performing caring work while carrying out bureaucratic mandates. Most scholarship recognizes that physical work is often prioritized over emotional care work in institutions (see for example James 1992), and strain occurs within the nursing profession between values of caring and bureaucracy (Davies 1995). Only a few studies have addressed the implications of home health nursing for the caregiver/nurse labor process (see Glazer 1993; Stone 2001; Ward-Griffin and Marshall 2003). Most work in home health has related to home health aides or home care aides (Eustis and Fischer 1991; Aronson and Neysmith 1996; Piercy and Dunkley 2004; Stacey 2005, 2011). This research shows that, particularly in light of cost-cutting measures, home health agencies also prioritize physical tasks (Aronson and Neysmith 1996), and aides' status as low-wage earners causes the potential for exploitation (Eustis and Fischer 1991). Aides may feel deep moral responsibilities to perform extra work (Aronson and Neysmith 1996), but strict rules mandated by legislation, credentialing processes, and payer sources often forbid them from performing skilled nursing care, and can cause them to struggle between what they know the patient needs and what they are allowed to do (Stone 2001; Stacey 2005, 2011).

11. As noted, Glazer's (1993) work sheds light on the structural reasons for the "work transfer" in nursing and retail. Drawing on Glazer (1984), Leidner's (1993) study of restaurant workers highlights the "work transfer" that occurs when customers must perform "voluntary unpaid labor"—such as standing in appropriate lines and gathering utensils. Much more work research is needed, however, regarding the interactional components of labor for caregivers engaged in skilled medical work at home.

12. A number of studies show that women's unpaid work serves to support public institutions and is often used to increase organizational functioning (Daniels 1987; DeVault 1991). Socialist feminists contend that "private sphere" activities include social reproduction that serves to uphold and maintain society—rearing children with a value system so that they become productive members of society, interfacing family members with social institutions such as schools, and providing emotional support (James 1989, 1992; Glazer 1993; Lorber 1994).

13. At that time, industrialization pulled men from their homes—then the centers of economic productivity—into factory work; women were left at home to assume household duties and care work (Coltrane and Galt 2000, 24–27; Padavic and Reskin 2002, 20–22). Protective labor laws enforced these changes by setting limits on women's hours and conditions of employment (Padavic and Reskin 2002, 22). Capitalist markets took over much of women's

former at-home craft and trade production (Coltrane and Galt 2000, 26). Popular media propagated this "cult of domesticity" by focusing on the sanctity and virtue of the home and women's rule over it (Abel 1991, 24–25). The illusions created by this ideology denied the social realities of single women, minorities, and working-class families in which women were still required to work for pay (DeVault 1991, 15; Glazer 1993, 29–32; Coltrane and Galt 2000, 27; Padavic and Reskin 2002, 24–26).

14. Economically and culturally, the function of "private sphere" work was to support a wage earner who was then free to enter the "public sphere" market (Kittay 1999). The private sphere work itself, however, has not been counted as part of society's "productive labor" (Folbre 2001). Illich (1981, 14) notes this difference when he describes the domestic labor of industrial societies as part of the "shadow economy," which functions to complement paid wage labor. See Macdonald (2010) for an analysis of childcare as "shadow" labor.

15. See Messias et al. (1997). See England (1992) for wage analyses of paid jobs considered "women's work." An analysis by England, Budig, and Folbre (2002) found that the wage penalty varied by occupation, and there was no penalty for nursing. According to an analysis by Howes, Leana, and Smith (2012, 72), we might expect the penalty to be greater for low-wage care workers than for high-wage "interactive" (face-to-face) care workers. See Folbre and Wright (2012, 4–5) for a complete definition of "interactive care work." See England (2005, 381) for theoretical frameworks for care work, including "devaluation," "public good," "prisoner of love," "commodification of emotion," and "love *and* money."

16. Studies show that women perform most of the housework (Coltrane 2000; Bittman and Wajcman 2000; Bittman et al. 2003), plan and obtain provisions for their families (DeVault 1991), and maintain social conversations and kinship ties (Fishman 1982; Di Leonardo 1992). Survey data from the National Alliance for Caregiving and the AARP show that 66 percent of the 65.7 million unpaid caregivers in the United States are women (NAC and AARP 2009, 14). Women are more likely to serve as primary caregivers, generally provide more "hands-on" care, and experience more stress in caregiving than do men (Horowitz 1985; also see Walker, Pratt, and Eddy 1995 for a review). In her analysis of research studies in Canada, Morris (2004, 106) finds that women feel greater obligations to perform unpaid care work, perform more demanding types of care, and travel greater distances to perform care. It is often women who are at an economic disadvantage due to their caregiving responsibilities (Baldwin and Glendinning 1983; Porterfield 2004; Wakabayashi and Donato 2006). Women caregivers are less likely to maintain formal labor market participation (Berecki-Gisolf et al. 2008), and when they begin caregiving early in life, they are at an increased disadvantage for poverty later on (Wakabayashi and Donato 2006).

17. The authors note that their definition of support care describes the tasks that Duffy (2005, 2011) has defined as "nonnurturant" care. Duffy (2005) has defined occupations as "nurturant" when they involve "face-to-face interaction and relationship with those being cared for," such as nurses, social workers, and teachers, and "nonnurturant" when they involve supportive services such as janitorial, food service, and administrative work (Duffy, Armenia, and Stacey 2015, 5). According to Duffy (2005, 2007), nonnurturant care jobs tend to have higher proportions of minority women.

18. See, for example, Gubrium and Sankar (1990).

19. In their study of eleven women caregivers of children with long-term care needs, geographers Yantzi and Rosenberg (2008) found that the caregivers experienced a disjuncture between the cultural ideal of home life and their daily life experiences.

20. Wiles (2003) interviewed caregivers of the elderly and found that "caregiving comes to dominate every experience; corporeal, emotional, social, and spatial" (1322). She finds that caregivers must deal with restricted mobility and often develop routines both to provide daily structure and to cope with all the tasks that must be done.

21. Prior research has shown that work performed in the private sphere has a multifaceted, shifting, and improvised nature, is often learned gradually and transmitted informally, and is frequently unacknowledged as "work" (Graham 1983; Daniels 1987; Smith 1987; DeVault 1991; James 1992).

22. This finding supports online survey results of 1,677 caregivers of primarily older adults, of whom 777 were performing nursing tasks, including helping with mobility devices and preparing special diets (Reinhard, Levine, and Samis 2012, 4). Results indicated that 73 percent of those who provided assistance with five or more medical/nursing tasks reported that their caregiving allowed family members to avoid being placed in a nursing home (32).

23. See manufacturing labor studies, for example Roy (1952); Braverman (1974); Burawoy (1979). See Folbre and Wright (2012) for their discussion of the importance of applying a labor process perspective to care work.

24. See Bowers (1990); Foner (1994), 113; Lindhardt, Bolmsjö, and Hallberg (2006).

25. Arras and Dubler (1995, 6) note that home care causes us to question our identities and social roles, and may involve inflicting pain on family members.

1. The Work Caregivers Do

1. Although I generally rely on Medicare definitions, the procedures that government agencies consider "skilled" reimbursable procedures may vary by state laws and change throughout time. For example, as discussed in chapter 3, Medicare no longer considers blood draws in the home to be skilled reimbursable procedures, unless they are performed in conjunction with other skilled procedures. I adopt a view that caregivers who are performing blood draws at home—as indeed one caregiver in this book is doing—are performing "skilled care" even though a home health nurse would not be reimbursed for this procedure unless it was performed in connection with another skilled procedure. See the appendix for a full discussion of the criteria used to select procedures.

2. I did not exclude caregivers based on any particular caregiving experience, occupation, or work history. A few said they had learned from prior experiences of taking care of family members, although that did not require the level of skilled care that they were currently performing. Nine caregivers had some current or prior experience in a health-related occupation. For example, two middle-aged caregivers had been nurses' aides for a short time around their high school years and believed their hands-on experience and the observation of nursing skills benefited them. Another had previously worked as a home health aide and believed the experience helped greatly because she had been able to observe nursing skills. Interestingly, two caregivers were registered nurses whose prior training was directly related to the medical procedures they performed, yet both discussed a variety of issues that made home medical care different for them, including the emotional component of caring for a family member, having to retool on certain tasks, and the malfunction of equipment at home.

3. This overview is intended for descriptive purposes only, and is not meant to endorse any particular procedure or protocol, nor should it be referred to as medical advice in the diagnosis or treatment of any medical disease or condition. For a comprehensive summary of the nursing procedures in home care, see Rice (2006a).

4. Central venous catheters (CVCs), such as Hickman-Broviac catheters or Groshong catheters, as well as implanted ports, are also used (Adams and Rice 2006, 385–91).

5. See Reinhard, Levine, and Samis (2012). In their survey of 1,677 caregivers, care recipients were generally elderly, with a mean age of seventy-one (13). The survey revealed that of the 373 caregivers who found medication management difficult, 110 of them, or 29 percent, reported being afraid of making a mistake or causing harm (24).

6. See Wolkowitz (2006) for further conceptualizations of body work.

2. On-the-Job Training

1. See Eitzen, Zinn, and Smith (2014) for a summary of the fragmentation and inefficiency in U.S. health care.

2. Workplace scholars have often looked at worker perceptions of status in understanding worker interactions. See, for example, Sherman (2007) for an interesting look at how luxury hotel workers recast their status in interacting with customers and clients.

3. When adult care recipients were available, and offered to tell me their viewpoints, they often talked about how they worked closely with caregivers to determine the best course of action in situations that required judgment.

4. This pattern was also noted in a study by Donelan et al. (2002).

5. The nursing literature is replete with articles about the importance of communication processes in discharge planning. For example, Wrobleski et al. (2014) find that bedside rounds are an effective approach.

3. Who Pays?

1. In 2009, at the time of my fieldwork, about 64 percent of Americans were covered by private health insurance and 31 percent were covered by Medicaid, Medicare, or military health care. About 17 percent, or approximately fifty million Americans, were uninsured (U.S. Census Bureau 2010). (Percentages do not sum to 100 as some Americans have multiple providers.) As of 2012, 63.9 percent had private health coverage, 32.6 percent were covered by government programs, and 15.4 percent were uninsured (U.S. Census Bureau 2013, 22).

2. About 65 percent of Medicaid beneficiaries nationally were enrolled in such plans as of 2006 (CMS 2007, 24).

3. The 1988 *Duggan v. Bowen* court case ruled in favor of a more liberal definition of "homebound," allowed for "part time or intermittent" services, and increased home health visits dramatically (Mayes and Berenson 2006, 99). According to Mayes and Berenson (2006, 99), between 1988 and 1995, home health care flourished and was the fastest-growing segment in the U.S. health care industry, experiencing a 168 percent increase in employment.

4. Balanced Budget Act of 1997, H.R. 2015, 105th Cong. (1997–1998), https://www.congress.gov/bill/105th-congress/house-bill/2015/text/enr.

5. As noted, skilled nursing services under Medicare must be "intermittent"—Medicare does not pay for twenty-four-hour coverage. Per my discussion with a home health administrator, as of 2009, during the period of my fieldwork, if there is a recurring intermittent need for skilled service (other than just drawing blood), "Medicare allows for twenty-one days of services or longer if there is a finite end point documented in the initial plan of care." Combined nursing and aide services "must be for less than eight hours a day, and twenty-eight hours per week." According to the administrator, following hospitalization, nursing and aide services can be provided for up to sixty days if the physician signs the appropriate discharge form. These sixty-day periods are called "sixty-day episodes" and can be renewed. Medicare does not pay for respite care for the caregiver. Medicare also covers hospice care when a doctor certifies that a patient is terminally ill and probably has less than six months to live, and the patient accepts palliative care (care for comfort instead of a cure) (CMS 2008, 38). This diagnosis can be recertified (38). Medicare pays for five days of inpatient respite care if the hospice staff determines it is needed. The patient pays 5 percent of the Medicare-approved cost for the hospital stay (38).

6. Medicare covers about 95 percent of the elderly population in the U.S., those of any age who have end-stage renal disease, and many people who are on Social Security disability (CMS 2007, 16; CMS 2008, 5). Parts A and B are most relevant to home care. Part A includes

hospital insurance and pays for inpatient hospital stays, home health, skilled nursing facilities, and hospice care. Part B covers physician bills, outpatient hospital bills, and home health and other services not covered by Part A. (Part A is free to most people who are Medicare eligible. Part B requires premium payments [CMS 2008, 5].) Part C is the Medicare Advantage program, which is administered by private health maintenance organizations (HMOs) or preferred provider organizations (PPOs) and often includes extra benefits for vision, dental, and prescription drugs (CMS 2008, 17, 60). Part D relates to prescription drug coverage. Because there are costs that Medicare doesn't cover, people often have supplemental coverage, such as a Medigap (Medicare Supplement Insurance) policy from a private insurer. These policies help cover costs of coinsurance, copayments, or deductibles (CMS 2008, 13). People with few resources can apply to their state programs for help and may qualify for state Medicaid. The latest data available, which pertained to the period of my fieldwork, are from 2008, at which time individuals had to have resources of $4,000 or less ($6,000 if married), and monthly income of less than $1,190 ($1,595 if married), in order to qualify. Individual states, however, vary on these amounts and may have higher limits (see CMS 2008, 14).

7. At the time of my fieldwork, approximately 56 percent of Americans on private insurance were in employer-based plans and about 9 percent were in direct-purchase plans (U.S. Census Bureau 2010). The most common type of employer-based plans were PPOs (57 percent of enrollees) and HMOs (21 percent of enrollees) (Kaiser 2008, 3). In PPOs, consumers are encouraged to choose physicians who are within a network of providers—the PPO itself does not actually provide health coverage. HMOs, on the other hand, serve as both insurers and direct providers or arrangers of care (2–4).

8. The National Association of Insurance Commissioners (NAIC) was established in 1871 to coordinate state insurance regulation, and the role of the states as primary regulators was officially codified in the 1945 McCarran-Ferguson Act (Kaiser 2008, 8; Jost 2009, 9). According to Kofman and Pollitz (2006, 5), state insurance departments regulate companies by requiring them to periodically file policies, and they also have the authority to conduct audits, issue fines or "cease and desist" orders, or revoke the licenses of companies that do not comply. Although regulation is largely in the hands of the states, according to policy experts, important federal laws regarding consumer protections do apply, including the Employee Retirement Income Security Act (ERISA) of 1974, the Consolidated Omnibus Budget Reconciliation Act of 1985 (COBRA), and the Health Insurance Portability and Accountability Act (HIPAA) of 1996 (Kofman and Pollitz 2006, 6; Kaiser 2008, 13–20). Both the states and the federal government enforce HIPAA, and most states have enacted laws that codify HIPAA protections; HIPAA leaves the regulation of premiums that may be charged for those with significant medical needs up to the states (Kofman and Pollitz 2006, 6). Under the federal 2010 ACA, premiums are capped based on income, and individuals and families may qualify to receive insurance subsidies. Beginning in 2014, the ACA banned discrimination based on preexisting conditions for adults (USDHHS 2018).

9. According to Kofman and Pollitz (2006, 3), in the small group market, although most states have enacted rate bands that limit premiums, as well as community rating, which requires that premiums be based on collective claims rather than claims for an individual, the state rating regulation rules vary significantly, and change with legislative actions.

10. The repeal becomes effective in 2019 (Eibner and Nowak 2018).

11. Under the Obama administration, these short-term policies were meant to be a "stopgap" measure and were limited to three months (Pear 2018).

12. According to Gornick, Howes, and Braslow (2012b, 141), many people who are eligible for services do not know that they are entitled to them: "Approximately half of uninsured children, for example, are eligible for public health insurance but their parents or guardians do not apply for it. . . . Those who do access publicly funded services often find that they are of poor quality."

13. Americans often envision a limited role for the state when it comes to health care (see Levitsky 2008). Yet surveys show that the majority favor established programs such as Medicaid and Medicare. According to the Pew Research Center, in 2011, a clear majority thought that Medicaid and Medicare have been "very good/good for the country" (Pew Research Center 2011). Although Obamacare initially received slightly negative or mixed reviews, in the wake of repeal and replace, its popularity rose, reaching 54 percent in February 2017 (Fingerhut 2017).

14. Discrimination against children who have preexisting medical conditions was made illegal in the 2010 Affordable Care Act—unfortunately this was too late for Hannah's son. As noted above, the ACA's ban on discrimination against adults with preexisting medical conditions went into effect in 2014.

15. In an interesting study by Stacey and Ayers (2012, 47), the authors found that family home care providers who were caring for disabled or elderly relatives, and who received an hourly wage under California's In-Home Supportive Services Program, perceived that such payment violated social norms, and thus framed their care work with an emphasis on skills and tasks and their contribution to the public good.

4. Integrating Care Work with Life

1. Lehoux, Saint-Arnaud, and Richard's (2004, 617) study of caregivers and care recipients showed that technology provides autonomy but also carries "heavy restrictions" and must be considered in light of the particular disease and the care recipient's life trajectory.

2. See Glenn (2010, 95–120) for historical legal case analyses of wives who had compensation agreements with their husbands or their husband's court-appointed guardian but were denied payment by the courts. Glenn also notes that Medicaid law has historically excluded "legally responsible relatives" from reimbursement for caregiving and states that allow for such compensation must "foot the entire cost" (115).

3. See Kane (1991) for a discussion of issues with home care organization, including fragmentation in delivery systems.

4. When Angus et al. (2005) studied households that received home care services in Ontario, they found that caregivers and care recipients had to make many adaptations to how their homes were arranged and organized. The caregivers in this book faced similar challenges.

5. Angus et al. found that those who could afford it were able to conceal health care equipment and supplies through storage options and other strategies, while those with fewer resources could not.

6. See also Angus et al. (2005, 176).

7. See Folbre (2012a, xii) for a discussion of the preference of care recipients (those with disabilities and the elderly) for consumer-directed home and community-based care, as opposed to institutional care.

8. See Corbin and Strauss (1988) for a discussion of how home health care reorders other work.

9. See Coltrane (2000). Women generally do more of the work that has a constant nature, such as cooking, cleaning, and laundry, while men "help out" or do less routine tasks such as taking out trash and doing yard work.

10. This bolsters Hochschild's finding that even when husbands help at home, women are more likely to feel responsible and to keep track of children, including their doctors' appointments (Hochschild with Machung 1989, 7).

11. Prior research demonstrates that extended family support can vary significantly by factors such as race, ethnicity, and socioeconomic class, with blacks and Latinos more likely to help extended family members with housework, childcare, and errands (Gerstel and Sarkisian 2008, 447). Gerstel and Sarkisian contend that much of the racial/ethnic differences are

related to socioeconomic class and the need for minority families to share resources (451). Much more work needs to be done to understand the sharing of tasks in the skilled labor process in minority and nontraditional families.

12. See Corbin and Strauss (1988, 112–14; 1990).

13. Corbin and Strauss (1990, 61) note this in their study of chronic illness. Their concept of the "making of arrangements" refers to "the process by which agreements are reached and maintained between persons for carrying out the tasks associated with home care."

14. See the introduction for citations regarding the nature of women's unpaid care work, and the likelihood and ideological underpinnings of women doing this type of work.

15. This does not mean, however, that men did not assume care in some cases. Hannah's father-in-law took early retirement and moved in to help so she could return to work and have more time to care for her other children. There were also a few cases in which aunts and uncles learned regular cystic fibrosis treatments for children, but primary caregivers generally administered all of the IVs. A few parents also said that the friends of their teenage or young adult children (who were care recipients) learned some of the procedures so they could spend more time with them. One caregiver actually had an organized schedule whereby church members (both women and men), including some RNs, came daily to help with skilled procedures—though this was an unusual circumstance.

16. See Daniels's (1987) discussion of the nature of women's work in maintaining everyday life, and Mayall (1993) for a discussion of Stacey and Davies's (1983) concept of the "intermediate domain." See England (1992), England, Budig, and Folbre (2002), and Howes, Leana, and Smith (2012) for their work on women in paid care professions.

17. See Bianchi, Folbre, and Wolf (2012) for a review of the literature.

18. See Bianchi, Folbre, and Wolf (2012) for a discussion of the issues facing single women in managing unpaid care work and paid employment.

19. This pattern reinforces Gerstel's (2000) notion of women's "third shift" of labor.

5. "You Do What You Gotta Do"

1. Folbre and Wright (2012, 6) note that although concern for a care recipient's well-being alone does not guarantee high-quality care, "it is *likely* to affect the quality of the services performed." Noddings (1995, 154) makes the point that we cannot assume what "people mean to each other" based only on their formal relationship. It is true that some caregivers may feel coerced or resent the assumption that they will care for family members (see Oliver 1983; Ungerson 1987, 46). Although the nurses I interviewed saw this dynamic, and would monitor care more closely, there is still much to learn about these situations as well as those in which caregivers do care but feel ill prepared or unable to carry out the skilled work.

2. Bolton (2000, 583) maintains that nurses can show kindness and professionalism without giving in to feelings of anger or sorrow, and referring to Lawler's (1991) work, she maintains that "nurses' skills in emotionally managing potentially awkward or embarrassing situations are a vital part of the caring process" (583).

3. In a detailed interdisciplinary review of the literature, Grandey, Diefendorff, and Rupp (2013, 5–6) maintain that emotional labor has been studied primarily through three lenses: *occupational requirements*, which are generally under the purview of sociology; *emotional displays*, which fall under organizational behavior; and *intrapsychic processes*, which generally fall under psychology. They conceptualize integration of these three theoretical lenses. Interestingly, the authors find that studies using current measurements have contradicted Hochschild's original claim that it is deep acting that most damages selfhood. These studies, according to the authors, have shown that "high surface acting is almost always more problematic than high deep acting" (16). The authors further note that the terms "emotion

management" and "emotion regulation" are used interchangeably with "emotion work" to "refer to modifying feelings and expressions in any context" (19).

4. The effect that caregiving has on the identity of caregivers is a complex issue. Medical sociologists have examined caregiver identity within the context of Bury's (1982) "biographical disruption." For example, Chamberlayne and King (1997, 605) cite Denzin's (1989, 23) work in which caregiving is seen as a "turning point in the biography, which significantly shapes the carer's life." Some caregivers are able to incorporate caregiving of the chronically ill into their preexisting identities, as well as their expectations for the future, while others experience dramatic changes. Caregivers have different emotional responses, coping mechanisms, resources, and opportunities. Further, caregivers are dealing with care recipients who have various illnesses, who are differentially related to them, and who have different senses of their own identities. Lawton (2003) points out that care recipients, while in danger of experiencing "biographical disruptions" that may inhibit their sense of hope for a normal future (Bury 1982) or a "loss of self" (Charmaz 1983), may also eventually be able to put their illness within a context from which they draw meaning (Williams 1984). These variances have profound effects on care recipients' identities and their relationships with caregivers, and influence caregivers' own sense of identity. While an extensive biographical analysis of care recipients' as well as caregivers' identities is beyond the scope of my analysis, what I aim to do in this chapter, through exploring the emotion work that caregivers perform, is to gain a greater understanding of how taking on skilled labor may affect caregivers' identities.

5. James refers to emotion work done in both the home and at paid jobs as "emotional labor," but I use Hochschild's term "emotion work" in this chapter.

6. It should be noted that prior work has suggested that caregivers may seek "outside help" in order to have more emotional detachment (Abel 1991, 113), but this did not appear to be an emotional mechanism used by the caregivers I interviewed. In cases where families eventually qualified for medical waivers, they had already experienced long periods of performing the procedures and/or were still performing a great many of them. Considering the intricate nature of the labor, its importance to life, and caregivers' part in it, it is more accurate to say that instead of "detachment," caregivers enacted "reattachment"—attaching to care recipients in new ways, with the relationship between them the central feature and driving force of their labor.

7. Care work scholars have noted the ideological importance of the marriage bond in caring relationships. According to Ungerson (1987, 51), "Marriage is regarded as the supreme caring relationship, rivalled perhaps only by the mother/infant bond." Corbin and Strauss (1988, 6) maintain that marriage carries the "weight of a legal and moral commitment." In response to Ungerson (1987), Glenn (2010, 90) notes that gendered familial relationships may influence spousal feelings of obligation toward ill spouses, as is the case when daughters or daughters-in-law provide care instead of husbands.

8. Interestingly, Murphy (1991), in a clinical study of stress and coping by caregivers of ventilator-dependent children, observed this same sentiment, which she identified as a coping strategy.

9. In a study performed in 2000, Williams demonstrated how mothers of teenage boys with a chronic illness act as "alert assistants" (Charmaz 1991, 69) in anticipating and meeting their sons' needs (Williams 2000, 254, 255). Williams (269) found that mothers acted in ways that minimized stigma so that sons could "pass successfully in public" (Goffman 1963), thus preserving their sense of masculinity (Charmaz 1995).

10. See also Stacey and Ayers (2012). Their interviews with paid family care providers for the elderly and disabled showed that caregivers believed others did not fully understand the scope of their work.

11. Granted, some commented that after they got used to the procedures, they could do them more quickly and without thinking—the labor became "like an old hat." Those with fewer procedures to perform may eventually feel that the work is very manageable. For example, one caregiver described taking care of an NG-tube as "nothing in my day."

12. Paid care workers also cite relationship as a reward for their interactions with clients. See, for example, Stacey's (2011) study of home care aides.

13. See Elmore (2014) for a review of findings regarding positive aspects of caring, including caregivers' sense of the importance of the work. Moreover, in *The Caring Self*, Stacey (2011, 96) notes that paid home care aides, while experiencing negative effects of the labor, such as frustration with families, also experience positive effects, including the ability to emotionally invest in their clients.

14. A national online survey by Reinhard, Levine, and Samis (2012, 7), of caregivers who were primarily taking care of older adults, showed that caregivers who were performing five or more medical/nursing tasks were more likely to report being close to the care recipient, and believed they were gaining new skills and making an important contribution. Yet compared to those performing only one to two tasks, they were also more likely to feel depressed, to feel that they constantly needed to watch for problems, to feel stressed about talking to many medical professionals, and to be worried about making a mistake.

15. See Green (2007, 159), who found that mothers caring for children with disabilities also felt that they were "stronger, better, more competent people with a greater appreciation for the important things in life and stronger, deeper relationships with friends and family."

16. Interestingly, newfound skills and knowledge directed some lay caregivers to seek careers in the medical profession. Even though she said she was not so originally inclined, one mother decided to attend nursing school and described her caregiving experiences as "the only reason I decided to do nursing." Family members from two other of the twenty-five families also chose careers in nursing because of their experiences.

17. See for example, Burton et al. (1997).

6. Work Shifts

1. Prior (2003, 48) estimates that the term "lay expert" has circulated through the medical sociology literature since at least the early 1990s, yet cautions that such "experiential knowledge" is limited, as caregivers lack the ability to diagnose and do not have access to multiple cases from which to frame their knowledge.

2. For example, as seen in chapter 4, several caregivers do not feel they receive direct evaluation once they are home.

3. In Great Britain, amid budget constraints, there is much current debate about the nursing profession, and nurses have been accused of not being caring enough. One critic even blamed feminism for the fact that nurses have tried to professionalize themselves to keep up with doctors and have, allegedly, lost the caring piece of their profession (Phillips 2011). Some critics argue that nursing has become so technical that the need for compassion has been overshadowed (Reed 2012).

4. Risman (2004, 1) argues that understanding gender "as a social structure" allows us to "better analyze the ways in which gender is embedded in the individual, interactional, and institutional dimensions of our society."

5. As seen in chapter 2, nurses do say they try to use a common language, or, as one told me, "put the skills into a context caregivers could understand." (This may be similar to Ward-Griffin and Marshall's [2003, 199] finding that nurses used a strategy of "describing skills in a simplistic way.")

6. See also Oudshoorn, Ward-Griffin, and McWilliam 2007. See also Theodosius's (2008, 42) discussion, which draws on Bolton and Boyd (2003), regarding the power that patients have as "consumers" or "customers."

7. These types of observations appear consistent with nursing scholarship on "primary nursing" (Porter 1992b; Smith 1991), which has advocated patient-centered versus task-centered labor processes (Bolton 2001, 91). Scholars refer to the "new nursing," or nursing practices that recognize a holistic and authentic relationship with the patient as an important component of nurses' labor (Bolton 2000, 581; Aldridge 1994; Smith 1991). See also Daykin and Clarke (2000, 354). This concept also emphasizes that patients/clients should be responsible for themselves—not "passive" or "'done to'" (Aldridge 1994, 724).

8. My findings are consistent with those of Luker et al. (2000, 776–8), who found that community palliative nurses in England felt they were better able to realize patients' "uniqueness," experience patient relationships, and "get to know the patient," thus achieving central components of the "new nursing" process. In Cain's (2015) study, hospice nurses also felt they could develop closer relationships with their patients, and enjoy quality time, leading to professional satisfaction (71, 72).

9. Prior research has shown the tension in bureaucracy, the worry that nurses have reduced time to care for patients, and the disjuncture between "holistic" nursing practices and the task processes that need to be accomplished in the hospital (Brannon 1994; Allen 2000; Daykin and Clarke 2000). Moreover, in institutions, caregivers who are engaged and ask lots of questions may slow down work processes for nurses (Brannon 1994). Allen (2000, 158), drawing on Salvage (1992), maintains that nurses who practice in hospitals face dilemmas because recognizing the expertise of family caregivers is crucial in "knowing the patient," yet doing so threatens to undermine nurses' professionalism.

10. Abel and Nelson (1990, 6) note that women perform similar caregiving activities in both public and private worlds, with tasks shifting back and forth between the two, and that events in one realm shape caregiving activities in the other.

11. Stacey (2011, 9) draws on work by Hochschild (2003, 203), who categorizes situations in which people are doing paid labor in other people's homes as "marketized private life." Marketized private life produces fuzzy feeling rules as workers negotiate between the expectations of employers and the private feeling rules of the home.

12. See Simmons, Nelson, and Neal's (2001) survey of RNs. Their analysis showed that home care nurses reported less frustration and anger with the system, less role ambiguity, and fewer workload conflicts than hospital nurses (69–71). Cain's (2015) study on hospice nurses showed that they, too, enjoyed the autonomy and flexibility of their work.

13. The importance of independent assessment by home health nurses is seen in a movement by the American Nurses Association. They have asked Congress to pass the Home Health Planning and Improvement Act, which would allow advanced practice registered nurses, nurse practitioners, and other nurse specialists to write orders for care plans and certification of home care services for Medicare patients (ANA 2012).

14. These findings are consistent with Stone (2001), who noted that nurses may pay extra visits or accept phone calls from patients even when they are at home.

Conclusion

1. See, for example, Glazer (1993).

2. As discussed in chapter 2, nurses maintain that caregivers must be "willing and able" to perform care. See Rice (2006b, 224) for an example of this language in the nursing literature.

3. See also work by Levine (2006, 2008), who argues for better ways to assess individual caregiver's abilities and willingness to take on the labor.

4. See Kittay (1999, 8–18).

5. The 2012 survey showed that caregivers needed more training in the complex medical tasks they were doing at home. See the introduction and chapter 2.

6. See Reinhard et al. (2019) for the complete findings and recommendations.

7. Stakeholders include hospital administrators, community and advocacy organizations, and caregivers. See Reinhard et al. (2019, 6–7) for methods.

8. See Reinhard et al. (2019, 7–8) for details.

9. These state caregiver programs include those in the National Family Caregiver Support Program (NFCSP), which is funded by federal grants through the Administration for Community Living (ACL).

10. See Avison et al. (2018) for evaluations of NFCSP programs. See Reinhard, Young, Levine, et al. (2019, 36) for recommendations regarding the need for comprehensive and proactive caregiver assessments that include cultural and generational factors.

11. See Gornick, Howes, and Braslow (2012b, 143–44) for critiques including restrictive definitions of family members, exclusion of employees who work in small businesses, lack of compliance, and the fact that lower-income employees are less likely to be aware of the law.

12. According to the National Partnership for Women and Families (NPWF), currently only four states—California, New Jersey, New York, and Rhode Island—have paid family leave programs, but such programs will begin in Washington and Massachusetts in 2019 and the District of Columbia in 2020 (NPWF 2019, 3).

13. See Folbre, Howes, and Leana (2012, 191–92) for models.

14. This amounts to two cents per ten dollars in wages (NPWF 2019, 1).

15. Social Security Caregiver Credit Act of 2017, S. 1255, 115th Cong., 1st Sess. (2017), https://www.congress.gov/115/bills/s1255/BILLS-115s1255is.pdf.

16. See ARCH (2019a) for respite networks.

17. The authors use the Zarit Burden Inventory (ZBI). See Zarit, Reever, and Bach-Peterson (1980).

18. The Mission Act of 2018 expanded the program to caregivers of veterans who incurred injury prior to 9/11, and is scheduled to begin after the VA certifies to Congress that it has implemented a required information technology system (USVA 2019d).

19. Although, as Levine (2008, 13) notes, hospice care has been more directed toward the family unit, and as stated, some state respite programs, as well as the VHA, have performed caregiver assessments.

20. The committee includes caregivers, providers, employers, veterans, older adults and individuals with disabilities, state and local officials, and others.

21. The act calls for a strategy that includes recommendations that are based on what federal, state, and local programs, health care providers, and long-term care services are doing, or can do, with respect to greater promotion of person- and family-centered care, assessment, education and training, respite, and financial security and workplace issues (AARP 2018). See Recognize, Assist, Include, Support, and Engage Family Caregivers Act of 2017, Pub. L. No. 115–119, 132 Stat. 23 (2018), https://www.congress.gov/115/plaws/publ119/PLAW-115publ119.pdf.

22. According to the 2019 *Home Alone Revisited* study, about 57 percent of participants felt they did not have a choice due to their own sense of responsibility as well as pressure from others (Reinhard, Young, Levine, et al. 2019, 33).

References

AARP. 2018. "RAISE Family Caregivers Act Now Law." Last updated October 15, 2019. https://www.aarp.org/politics-society/advocacy/caregiving-advocacy/info-2015/raise-family-caregivers-act.html.

AARP. 2019. "Can I Get Paid to Be a Caregiver for a Family Member?" Last updated October 15, 2019. https://www.aarp.org/caregiving/financial-legal/info-2017/you-can-get-paid-as-a-family-caregiver.html.

ACL (Administration for Community Living). 2019a. "Lifespan Respite Care Program." https://acl.gov/programs/support-caregivers/lifespan-respite-care-program.

ACL (Administration for Community Living). 2019b. "National Family Caregiver Support Program." https://acl.gov/programs/support-caregivers/national-family-caregiver-support-program.

ADA (American Diabetes Association). 2011. "Insulin Pumps." http://www.diabetes.org/living-with-diabetes/treatment-and-care/medication/insulin/insulin-pumps.html (site discontinued).

ANA (American Nurses Association). 2012. "Home Health Planning and Improvement Act." http://www.rnaction.org/homehealth (site discontinued).

ARCH (National Respite Network and Resource Center). 2019a. ARCH website. https://archrespite.org.

ARCH (National Respite Network and Resource Center). 2019b. "Lifespan Respite Reauthorization Center." https://archrespite.org/national-respite-coalition/reauthorize-lifespan-respite.

AUAF (American Urological Association Foundation). 2010. "Managing Bladder Dysfunction with Products and Devices." http://www.urologyheatlh.org/adult/index.cfm?cat=03&topic=390 (site discontinued).

Abel, Emily K. 1991. *Who Cares for the Elderly? Public Policy and the Experiences of Adult Daughters.* Philadelphia: Temple University Press.

Abel, Emily K., and Margaret K. Nelson. 1990. "Circles of Care: An Introductory Essay." In *Circles of Care: Work and Identity in Women's Lives*, edited by Emily K. Abel and Margaret K. Nelson, 4–34. Albany: State University of New York Press.

Acker, Joan. 1990. "Hierarchies, Jobs, Bodies: A Theory of Gendered Organizations." *Gender & Society* 4 (2): 139–58.

Adams, Sally C., and Robyn Rice. 2006. "The Patient Receiving Home Infusion Therapies." In Rice, *Home Care Nursing Practice*, 381–402.

Ahmann, Elizabeth, with revisions by Virginia C. Gebus. 1996. "Home Care of the Infant or Child Requiring Tube Feeding." In *Home Care for the High-Risk Infant: A Family-Centered Approach*, edited by Elizabeth Ahmann, 135–49. Gaithersburg MD: Aspen.

Ahmann, Elizabeth, with revisions by Angela Jerome-Ebel. 1996. "Home Care of the Infant Requiring Mechanical Ventilation." In *Home Care for the High-Risk Infant: A Family-Centered Approach*, edited by Elizabeth Ahmann, 235–49. Gaithersburg, MD: Aspen.

Ahmann, Elizabeth, with revisions by Dorothy Page. 1996. "Home Care of the Infant with Respiratory Compromise." In *Home Care for the High-Risk Infant: A Family-Centered Approach*, edited by Elizabeth Ahmann, 171–82. Gaithersburg MD: Aspen.

Albert, Steven M. 1990. "The Dependent Elderly, Home Health Care, and Strategies of Household Adaptation." In *The Home Care Experience: Ethnography and Policy*, edited by Jaber F. Gubrium and Andrea Sankar, 19–36. Newbury Park, CA: Sage.

Aldridge, Meryl. 1994. "Unlimited Liability? Emotional Labour in Nursing and Social Work." *Journal of Advanced Nursing* 20:722–28.

Allan, Graham, and Graham Crow. 1989. Introduction to *Home and Family: Creating the Domestic Sphere*, edited by Graham Allan and Graham Crow, 1–13. London: Macmillan.

Allen, Davina. 2000. "Negotiating the Role of Expert Carers on an Adult Hospital Ward." *Sociology of Health & Illness* 22 (2): 149–71.

Angus, Jan. 1994. "Women's Paid/Unpaid Work and Health: Exploring the Social Context of Everyday Life." *Canadian Journal of Nursing Research* 26 (4): 23–42.

Angus, Jan, Pia Kontos, Isabel Dyck, Patricia McKeever, and Blake Poland. 2005. "The Personal Significance of Home: Habitus and the Experience of Receiving Long-Term Home Care." *Sociology of Health & Illness* 27 (2): 161–87.

Aronson, Jane, and Sheila M. Neysmith. 1996. "'You're Not Just in There to Do the Work': Depersonalizing Policies and the Exploitation of Home Care Workers' Labor." *Gender & Society* 10 (1): 59–77.

Arras, John D., and Nancy Neveloff Dubler. 1995. "Ethical and Social Implications of High-Tech Home Care." In *Bringing the Hospital Home: Ethical and Social Implications of High-Tech Home Care*, edited by John D. Arras, 1–31. Baltimore: Johns Hopkins University Press.

Avison, Cecilia, Dwight Brock, Joanne Campione, Susan Hassell, Beth Rabinovich, Robin Ritter, Jacqueline Severynse, Duck-Hye Yang, and Katarzyna Zebrak. 2018. *Outcome Evaluation of the National Family Caregiver Support Program*. Washington, DC: Administration for Community Living. December 5, 2018. https://acl.gov/sites/default/files/programs/2018-12/Caregiver_Outcome_Evaluation_Final_Report.pdf.

Baldwin, Sally, and Caroline Glendinning. 1983. "Employment, Women and Their Disabled Children." In *A Labour of Love: Women, Work and Caring*, edited by Janet Finch and Dulcie Groves, 53–71. London: Routledge and Kegan Paul.

Berecki-Gisolf, Janneke, Jayne Lucke, Richard Hockey, and Annette Dobson. 2008. "Transitions into Informal Caregiving and Out of Paid Employment of Women in Their 50s." *Social Science and Medicine* 67 (1): 122–27.

Bianchi, Suzanne, Nancy Folbre, and Douglas Wolf. 2012. "Unpaid Care Work." In *For Love and Money: Care Provision in the United States*, edited by Nancy Folbre, 40–64. New York: Russell Sage Foundation.

Bittman, Michael, Paula England, Liana Sayer, Nancy Folbre, and George Matheson. 2003. "When Does Gender Trump Money? Bargaining and Time in Household Work." *American Journal of Sociology* 109 (1): 186–214.

Bittman, Michael, and Judy Wajcman. 2000. "The Rush Hour: The Character of Leisure Time and Gender Equity." *Social Forces* 79 (1): 165–89.

Boland, Donna L., and Sharon L. Sims. 1996. "Family Caregiving at Home as a Solitary Journey." *Journal of Nursing Scholarship* 28 (1): 55–58.

Bolton, Sharon C. 2000. "Who Cares? Offering Emotions Work as a 'Gift' in the Nursing Labour Process." *Journal of Advanced Nursing* 32 (3): 580–86.

Bolton, Sharon C. 2001. "Changing Faces: Nurses as Emotional Jugglers." *Sociology of Health & Illness* 23 (1): 85–100.

Bolton, Sharon C., and Carol Boyd. 2003. "Trolley Dolly or Skilled Emotion Manager? Moving on from Hochschild's Managed Heart." *Work, Employment and Society* 17 (2): 289–308.

Boris, Eileen, and Jennifer Klein. 2012. *Caring for America: Home Health Workers in the Shadow of the Welfare State*. Oxford: Oxford University Press.

Bourdieu, Pierre. 1977. *Outline of a Theory of Practice*. Cambridge: Cambridge University Press.

Bourdieu, Pierre. 1990a. *In Other Words: Essays toward a Reflexive Sociology*. Stanford, CA: Stanford University Press.

Bourdieu, Pierre. 1990b. *The Logic of Practice*. Stanford, CA: Stanford University Press.

Bowers, Barbara. 1990. "Family Perceptions of Care in a Nursing Home." In *Circles of Care: Work and Identity in Women's Lives*, edited by Emily K. Abel and Margaret K. Nelson, 278–89. Albany: State University of New York Press.

Brannon, Robert L. 1994. "Professionalization and Work Intensification: Nursing in the Cost Containment Era." *Work and Occupations* 21 (2): 157–78.

Braverman, Harry. 1974. *Labor and Monopoly Capital: The Degradation of Work in the Twentieth Century*. New York: Monthly Review Press.

Brown, Stephanie L., Dylan M. Smith, Richard Schulz, Mohammed U. Kabeto, Peter A. Ubel, Michael Poulin, Jayhee Yi, Catherine Kim, and Kenneth M. Langa. 2009. "Caregiving Behavior Is Associated with Decreased Mortality Risk." *Psychological Science* 20 (4): 488–94. https://doi.org/10.1111/j.1467-9280.2009.02323.x.

Bunce, Victoria Craig, and J. P. Wieske. 2009. *Health Insurance Mandates in the States 2009*. Alexandria, VA: Council for Affordable Health Insurance. https://www2.cbia.com/ieb/ag/CostOfCare/RisingCosts/CAHI_HealthInsuranceMandates2009.pdf.

Burawoy, Michael. 1979. *Manufacturing Consent: Changes in the Labor Process under Monopoly Capitalism*. Chicago: University of Chicago Press.

Burton, L. C., J. T. Newsom, R. Schulz, C. H. Hirsch, and P. S. German. 1997. "Preventative Health Behaviors among Spousal Caregivers." *Preventative Medicine* 26 (2): 162–69.

Bury, Michael. 1982. "Chronic Illness as Biographical Disruption." *Sociology of Health & Illness* 4 (2): 167–82.

Cain, Cindy L. 2015. "Orienting End of Life Care: The Hidden Value of Hospice Home Visits." In *Caring on the Clock: The Complexities and Contradictions of Paid Care Work*, edited by Mignon Duffy, Amy Armenia, and Clare L. Stacey, 67–81. New Brunswick, NJ: Rutgers University Press.

Cancian, Francesca M. 2000. "Paid Emotional Care: Organizational Forms That Encourage Nurturance." In *Care Work: Gender, Labor and the Welfare State*, edited by Madonna Harrington Meyer, 136–48. New York: Routledge.

Cancian, Francesca M., and Stacey J. Oliker. 2000. *Caring and Gender*. Walnut Creek, CA: Alta Mira.

Cannuscio, C. C., G. A. Colditz, E. B. Rimm, L. F. Berkman, C. P. Jones, and I. Kawachi. 2004. "Employment Status, Social Ties, and Caregivers' Mental Health." *Social Science & Medicine* 58 (7): 1247–56.

CBO (Congressional Budget Office). 2007. *The Long-Term Outlook for Health Care Spending*. Washington, DC: Congressional Budget Office. November 2007. https://www.cbo.gov/sites/default/files/110th-congress-2007-2008/reports/11-13-lt-health.pdf.

Chamberlayne, Prue, and Annette King. 1997. "The Biographical Challenge of Caring." *Sociology of Health & Illness* 19 (5): 601–21.

Chambliss, Daniel F. 1996. *Beyond Caring: Hospitals, Nurses, and the Social Organization of Ethics*. Chicago: University of Chicago Press.

Charmaz, Kathy. 1983. "Loss of Self: A Fundamental Form of Suffering in the Chronically Ill." *Sociology of Health & Illness* 5 (2): 168–95.

Charmaz, Kathy. 1991. *Good Days, Bad Days: The Self in Chronic Illness and Time*. New Brunswick, NJ: Rutgers University Press.

Charmaz, Kathy. 1995. "Identity Dilemmas of Chronically Ill Men." In *Men's Health and Illness: Gender, Power, and the Body*, edited by Donald F. Sabo and David Frederick Gordon, 266–91. Thousand Oaks, CA: Sage.

CLTC (Commission on Long-Term Care). 2013. *Report to the Congress*. Washington, DC: Government Printing Office. September 30, 2013. https://www.govinfo.gov/content/pkg/GPO-LTCCOMMISSION/pdf/GPO-LTCCOMMISSION.pdf.

CMS (Centers for Medicare and Medicaid Services). 2007. *Brief Summaries of Medicare and Medicaid: Title XVIII and Title XIX of the Social Security Act as of*

November 1, 2007. Prepared by Earl Dirk Hoffman Jr., Barbara S. Klees, and Catherine A Curtis, Office of the Actuary. Baltimore: CMS. https://www.cms.gov/Research-Statistics-Data-and-Systems/Research/MedicareMedicaidStatSupp/Downloads/07BriefSummaries.pdf.

CMS (Centers for Medicare and Medicaid Services). 2008. *Your Medicare Benefits*. CMS Publication No. 10116. Baltimore: U.S. Department of Health and Human Services.

CMS (Centers for Medicare and Medicaid Services). 2010a. *Home Health PPS Overview*. Baltimore: CMS. http://www.cms.gov/HomeHealthPPS/.

CMS (Centers for Medicare and Medicaid Services). 2010b. *Medicare and Home Health Care*. Baltimore: CMS. https://www.medicare.gov/Pubs/pdf/10969-Medicare-and-Home-health-Care.pdf.

Coltrane, Scott. 2000. "Research on Household Labor: Modeling and Measuring the Social Embeddedness of Routine Family Work." *Journal of Marriage and the Family* 62 (4): 1208–33.

Coltrane, Scott, and Justin Galt. 2000. "The History of Men's Caring: Evaluating Precedents for Fathers' Family Involvement." In *Care Work: Gender, Labor and the Welfare State*, edited by Madonna Harrington Meyer, 15–36. New York: Routledge.

Corbin, Juliet M., and Anselm Strauss. 1988. *Unending Work and Care: Managing Chronic Illness at Home*. San Francisco: Jossey-Bass.

Corbin, Juliet M., and Anselm Strauss. 1990. "Making Arrangements: The Key to Home Care." In *The Home Care Experience: Ethnography and Policy*, edited by Jaber F. Gubrium and Andrea Sankar, 59–73. Newbury Park, CA: Sage.

Cuba, Lee, and David M. Hummon. 1993. "A Place to Call Home: Identification with Dwelling, Community, and Region." *Sociological Quarterly* 34 (1): 111–31.

Daniels, Arlene Kaplan. 1987. "Invisible Work." *Social Problems* 34 (5): 403–15.

Davies, Celia. 1995. "Competence versus Care? Gender and Caring Work Revisited." *Acta Sociologica* 38:17–31.

Day, Jennifer R., and Ruth A. Anderson. 2011. "Compassion Fatigue: An Application of the Concept to Informal Caregivers of Family Members with Dementia." *Nursing Research and Practice* 2011:1–10.

Daykin, Norma, and Brenda Clarke. 2000. " 'They'll Still Get the Bodily Care': Discourses of Care and Relationships between Nurses and Health Care Assistants in the NHS." *Sociology of Health & Illness* 22 (3): 349–63.

Denzin, Norman. 1989. *Interpretive Biography*. London: Sage.

DeVault, Marjorie. L. 1991. *Feeding the Family: The Social Organization of Caring as Gendered Work*. Chicago: University of Chicago Press.

DeVault, Marjorie. L. 1999. "Comfort and Struggle: Emotion Work in Family Life." In *Emotional Labor in the Service Economy: The Annals of the American Academy of Political and Social Sciences*, edited by Ronnie J. Steinberg and Deborah M. Figart, 52–63. Thousand Oaks, CA: Sage.

Di Leonardo, Michaela. 1992. "The Female World of Cards and Holidays: Women, Families, and the Work of Kinship." In *Rethinking the Family: Some Feminist Questions*, edited by Barrie Thorne and Marilyn Yalom, 246–61. Boston: Northeastern University Press.

Diamond, Timothy. 1992. *Making Gray Gold: Narratives of Nursing Home Care*. Chicago: University of Chicago Press.

Doerner, William G., and Steven P. Lab. 2015. *Victimology*. 7th ed. Waltham, MA: Anderson/Elsevier.

Donelan, Karen, Craig A. Hill, Catherine Hoffman, Kimberly Scoles, Penny Hollander Feldman, Carol Levine, and David Gould. 2002. "Challenged to Care: Informal Caregivers in a Changing Health System." *Health Affairs* 21 (4): 222–31.

Driscoll, Colette Duncliffe. 1996. "Home Care of the Infant or Child with a Tracheostomy." In *Home Care for the High-Risk Infant: A Family-Centered Approach*, edited by Elizabeth Ahmann, 221–34. Gaithersburg, MD: Aspen.

Duffy, Mignon. 2005. "Reproducing Labor Inequalities: Challenges for Feminists Conceptualizing Care at the Intersections of Gender, Race, and Class." *Gender & Society* 19 (1): 66–82.

Duffy, Mignon. 2007. "Doing the Dirty Work: Gender, Race, and Reproductive Labor in Historical Perspective." *Gender & Society* 21 (3): 313–36.

Duffy, Mignon. 2011. *Making Care Count: A Century of Gender, Race, and Paid Care Work*. New Brunswick, NJ: Rutgers University Press.

Duffy, Mignon, Randy Albelda, and Clare Hammonds. 2013. "Counting Care Work: The Empirical and Policy Applications of Care Theory." *Social Problems* 60 (2): 145–67.

Duffy, Mignon, Amy Armenia, and Clare L. Stacey. 2015. "On the Clock, off the Radar." In *Caring on the Clock: The Complexities and Contradictions of Paid Care Work*, edited by Mignon Duffy, Amy Armenia, and Clare L. Stacey, 3–13. New Brunswick, NJ: Rutgers University Press.

Duffy, Mignon, Clare L. Stacey, and Amy Armenia. 2015. "Making Paid Care Work." In *Caring on the Clock: The Complexities and Contradictions of Paid Care Work*, edited by Mignon Duffy, Amy Armenia, and Clare L. Stacey, 287–91. New Brunswick, NJ: Rutgers University Press.

Edwards, Carol, Sophie Staniszweska, and Nicola Crichton. 2004. "Investigation of the Ways in Which Patients' Reports of Their Satisfaction with Healthcare Are Constructed." *Sociology of Health & Illness* 26 (2): 159–83.

Eibner, Christine, and Sarah A. Nowak. 2018. "The Effect of Eliminating the Individual Mandate Penalty and the Role of Behavioral Factors." Commonwealth Fund, July 11, 2018. https://www.commonwealthfund.org/publications/fund-reports/2018/jul/eliminating-individual-mandate-penalty-behavioral-factors.

Eitzen, D. Stanley, Maxine Baca Zinn, and Kelly Eitzen Smith. 2014. "The Healthcare System." In *Social Problems*, 430–58. London: Pearson.

Elmore, Diane L. 2014. "The Impact of Caregiving on Physical and Mental Health: Implications for Research, Practice, Education and Policy." In *The Challenges of Mental Health Caregiving: Research, Practice, Policy*, edited by Rhonda C. Talley, Gregory L. Fricchione, and Benjamin G. Druss, 15–31. New York: Springer-Verlag.

England, Kim, and Isabel Dyck. 2011. "Managing the Body Work of Home Care." *Sociology of Health & Illness* 33 (2): 206–19.

England, Paula. 1992. *Comparable Worth: Theories and Evidence*. New York: Walter De Gruyter.

England, Paula. 2005. "Emerging Theories of Care Work." *Annual Review of Sociology* 31:381–99.

England, Paula, Michelle Budig, and Nancy Folbre. 2002. "Wages of Virtue: The Relative Pay of Care Work." *Social Problems* 49 (4): 455–73.

England, Paula, Nancy Folbre, and Carrie Leana. 2012. "Motivating Care." In *For Love and Money: Care Provision in the United States*, edited by Nancy Folbre, 21–39. New York: Russell Sage Foundation.

Erickson, Rebecca J. 1993. "Reconceptualizing Family Work: The Effect of Emotion Work on Perceptions of Marital Quality." *Journal of Marriage and the Family* 55:888–900.

Erickson, Rebecca J. 2005. "Why Emotion Work Matters: Sex, Gender, and the Division of Household Labor." *Journal of Marriage and Family* 67:337–51.

Erickson, Rebecca J. 2011. "Emotional Carework, Gender, and the Division of Household Labor." In *At the Heart of Work and Family: Engaging the Ideas of Arlie Hochschild*, edited by Anita Ilta Garey and Karen V. Hansen, 61–73. New Brunswick, NJ: Rutgers University Press.

Erickson, Rebecca J., and Clare L. Stacey. 2013. "Attending to Mind and Body: Engaging the Complexity of Emotion Practice among Caring Professionals." In *Emotional Labor in the 21st Century: Diverse Perspectives on Emotion Regulation at Work*, edited by Alicia A. Grandey, James M. Diefendorff, and Deborah E. Rupp, 175–96. New York: Routledge.

Eustis, Nancy N., and Lucy Rose Fischer. 1991. "Relationships between Home Care Clients and Their Workers: Implications for Quality of Care." *Gerontologist* 31 (4): 447–56.

Feinberg, Lynn, Susan C. Reinhard, Ari Houser, and Rita Choula. 2011. *Valuing the Invaluable: 2011 Update; The Growing Contributions and Costs of Family Caregiving*. Washington, DC: AARP Public Policy Institute. http://assets.aarp.org/rgcenter/ppi/ltc/i51-caregiving.pdf.

Fingerhut, Hannah. 2017. "Support for 2010 Health Care Law Reaches New High." Pew Research Center, February 23, 2017. http://www.pewresearch.org/fact-tank/2017/02/23/support-for-2010-health-care-law-reaches-new-high/.

Fisher, Berenice, and Tronto, Joan. 1990. "Toward a Feminist Theory of Caring." In *Circles of Care: Work and Identity in Women's Lives*, edited by Emily K. Abel and Margaret K. Nelson, 35–62. Albany: State University of New York Press.

Fishman, Pamela. 1982. "Interaction: The Work Women Do." In *Women and Work: Problems and Perspectives*, edited by Rachel Kahn-Hut, Arlene Kaplan Daniels, and Richard Colvard, 170–201. New York: Oxford University Press.

Folbre, Nancy. 2001. *The Invisible Heart: Economics and Family Values*. New York: New Press.

Folbre, Nancy. 2012a. Introduction to *For Love and Money: Care Provision in the United States*, edited by Nancy Folbre, xi–xvii. New York: Russell Sage Foundation.

Folbre, Nancy. 2012b. "Valuing Care." In *For Love and Money: Care Provision in the United States*, edited by Nancy Folbre, 92–111. New York: Russell Sage Foundation.

Folbre, Nancy, Candace Howes, and Carrie Leana. 2012. "A Care Policy and Research Agenda." In *For Love and Money: Care Provision in the United States*, edited by Nancy Folbre, 183–204. New York: Russell Sage Foundation.

Folbre, Nancy, and Erik Olin Wright. 2012. "Defining Care." In *For Love and Money: Care Provision in the United States*, edited by Nancy Folbre, 1–20. New York: Russell Sage Foundation.

Foner, Nancy. 1994. *The Caregiving Dilemma: Work in an American Nursing Home*. Berkeley: University of California Press.

Frey, Allison, Stephanie Mika, Rachel Nuzum, and Cathy Schoen. 2009. "Setting a National Standard for Health Benefits: How Do State Benefit Mandates Compare with Benefits in Large-Group Plans?" Commonwealth Fund, pub. 1292, vol. 56.

Gerstel, Naomi. 2000. "The Third Shift: Gender and Care Work outside the Home." *Qualitative Sociology* 23 (4): 467–83.

Gerstel, Naomi, and Natalia Sarkisian. 2008. "The Color of Family Ties: Race, Class, Gender, and Extended Family Involvement." In *American Families: A Multicultural Reader*, 2nd ed., edited by Stephanie Coontz with Maya Parson and Gabrielle Raley, 447–53. New York: Routledge.

Giddens, Anthony. 1977. *Studies in Social and Political Theory*. London: Hutchinson.

Giddens, Anthony. 1984. *The Constitution of Society: Outline of the Theory of Structuration*. Cambridge: Polity.

Gimlin, Debra. 2007. "What Is 'Body Work'? A Review of the Literature." *Sociology Compass* 1 (1): 353–70.

Glazer, Nona Y. 1984. "Servants to Capital: Unpaid Domestic Labor and Paid Work." *Review of Radical Political Economics* 16:61–87.

Glazer, Nona Y. 1990. "The Home as Workshop: Women as Amateur Nurses and Medical Care Providers." *Gender & Society* 4 (4): 479–99.

Glazer, Nona Y. 1993. *Women's Paid and Unpaid Labor: The Work Transfer in Health Care and Retailing*. Philadelphia: Temple University Press.

Glenn, Evelyn Nakano. 2000. "Creating a Caring Society." *Contemporary Sociology* 29 (1): 84–94.

Glenn, Evelyn Nakano. 2010. *Forced to Care: Coercion and Caregiving in America*. Cambridge, MA: Harvard University Press.

Goffman, Erving. 1963. *Stigma*. Englewood Cliffs, NJ: Prentice Hall.

Goodman, Ellen. 2008. "The Do-It-Yourself Economy." AlterNet, July 18, 2008. http://www.alternet.org/story/91872/the_do-it-yourself_economy.

Gordon, Suzanne. 2006. "The New Cartesianism: Dividing Mind and Body and Thus Disembodying Care." In *The Complexities of Care: Nursing Reconsidered*, edited by Sioban Nelson and Suzanne Gordon, 104–21. Ithaca, NY: Cornell University Press.

Gordon, Suzanne. 2017. *The Battle for Veterans' Healthcare: Dispatches from the Frontlines of Policy Making and Patient Care*. Ithaca, NY: Cornell University Press.

Gordon, Suzanne, and Sioban Nelson. 2006. "Moving beyond the Virtue Script in Nursing: Creating a Knowledge-Based Identity for Nurses." In *The Complexities of Care: Nursing Reconsidered*, edited by Sioban Nelson and Suzanne Gordon, 13–29. Ithaca, NY: Cornell University Press.

Gornick, Janet, Candace Howes, and Laura Braslow. 2012a. "The Care Policy Landscape." In *For Love and Money: Care Provision in the United States*, edited by Nancy Folbre, 112–39. New York: Russell Sage Foundation.

Gornick, Janet, Candace Howes, and Laura Braslow. 2012b. "The Disparate Impacts of Care Policy." In *For Love and Money: Care Provision in the United States*, edited by Nancy Folbre, 140–82. New York: Russell Sage Foundation.

Graham, Hilary. 1983. "Caring: A Labour of Love." In *A Labour of Love: Women, Work and Caring*, edited by Janet Finch and Dulcie Groves, 13–30. London: Routledge and Kegan Paul.

Grandey, Alicia A., James M. Diefendorff, and Deborah E. Rupp. 2013. "Bringing Emotional Labor into Focus: A Review and Integration of Three Research Lenses." In *Emotional Labor in the 21st Century: Diverse Perspectives on Emotion Regulation at Work*, edited by Alicia A. Grandey, James M. Diefendorff, and Deborah E. Rupp, 3–27. New York: Routledge.

Green, Sara Eleanor. 2007. " 'We're Tired, Not Sad': Benefits and Burdens of Mothering a Child with a Disability." *Social Science and Medicine* 64:150–63.

Guberman, Nancy, Éric Gagnon, Denyse Côté, Claude Gilbert, Nicole Thivièrge, and Marielle Tremblay. 2005. "How the Trivialization of the Demands of High-Tech Care in the Home Is Turning Family Members into Para-Medical Personnel." *Journal of Family Issues* 26 (2): 247–72.

Gubrium, Jaber F., and Andrea Sankar. 1990. Introduction to *The Home Care Experience: Ethnography and Policy*, edited by Jaber F. Gubrium and Andrea Sankar, 7–15. Newbury Park, CA: Sage.

Heaton, Janet. 1999. "The Gaze and Visibility of the Carer: A Foucauldian Analysis of the Discourse of Informal Care." *Sociology of Health & Illness* 21 (6): 759–77.

Hirst, M. 2005. "Carer Distress: A Prospective, Population-Based Study." *Social Science & Medicine* 61 (3): 697–708.

Hochschild, Arlie Russell. 1979. "Emotion Work, Feelings Rules, and Social Structure." *American Journal of Sociology* 85:551–75.

Hochschild, Arlie Russell. 1983. *The Managed Heart: Commercialization of Human Feeling*. Berkeley: University of California Press.

Hochschild, Arlie Russell. 2003. *The Managed Heart: Commercialization of Human Feeling*. 20th anniversary ed. Berkeley: University of California Press.

Hochschild, Arlie Russell, with Anne Machung. 1989. *The Second Shift: Working Parents and the Revolution at Home*. New York: Viking.

Hodson, Randy. 2001. *Dignity at Work*. Cambridge: Cambridge University Press.

hooks, bell. 1987. "Feminism: A Movement to End Sexist Oppression." In *Equality and Feminism*, edited by Anne Phillips, 62–76. New York: NYU Press.

Horowitz, Amy. 1985. "Sons and Daughters as Caregivers to Older Parents: Differences in Role Performance and Consequences." *Gerontologist* 25 (6): 612–17.

Houston, Kathryn A. 2006. "The Patient with Bladder Dysfunction." In Rice, *Home Care Nursing Practice*, 281–300.

Howes, Candace, Carrie Leana, and Kristin Smith. 2012. "Paid Care Work." In *For Love and Money: Care Provision in the United States*, edited by Nancy Folbre, 65–91. New York: Russell Sage Foundation.

I-Flow Corporation. 2011. "Homepump Eclipse® Infusion System." http://www.iflo.com/prod_homepump.php (site discontinued).

Illich, Ivan. 1981. *Shadow Work*. Boston: Marion Boyars.

James, Nicky. 1989. "Emotional Labour: Skill and Work in the Social Regulation of Feelings." *Sociological Review* 37 (1): 15–42.

James, Nicky. 1992. "Care = Organization + Physical Labour + Emotional Labour." *Sociology of Health & Illness* 14 (4): 488–509.

Jaudes, Paula Kienberger. 1991. "The Medical Care of Children with Complex Home Health Care Needs: An Overview for Caretakers." In *The Medically Complex Child: The Transition to Home Care*, edited by Neil J. Hochstadt and Diane M. Yost, 29–60. Chur, Switzerland: Harwood Academic.

Jost, Timothy Stoltzfus. 2009. "The Regulation of Private Health Insurance." Social Science Research Network, January 30, 2009. https://doi.org/10.2139/ssrn.1340092.

Kaiser (Henry J. Kaiser Family Foundation). 2008. *How Private Health Coverage Works: A Primer; 2008 Update*. April 2008. Menlo Park, CA: Henry J. Kaiser Family Foundation. http://www.kff.org/insurance/upload/7766.pdf.

Kaiser (Henry J. Kaiser Family Foundation). 2019. "Status of State Medicaid Expansion Decisions: Interactive Map." November 6, 2019. https://www.kff.org/medicaid/issue-brief/status-of-state-medicaid-expansion-decisions-interactive-map/.

Kane, Rosalie A. 1991. "High-Tech Home Care in Context." In *Bringing the Hospital Home: Ethical and Social Implications of High-Tech Home Care*, edited by John D. Arras, 197–219. Baltimore: Johns Hopkins University Press.

Kittay, Eva Feder. 1999. *Love's Labor: Essays on Women, Equality, and Dependency*. New York: Routledge.

Kofman, Mila, and Karen Pollitz. 2006. *Health Insurance Regulation by States and the Federal Government: A Review of Current Approaches and Proposals for Change*. Washington, DC: Georgetown University Health Policy Institute. April 2006. https://www-tc.pbs.org/now/politics/Healthinsurancereportfinalkofmanpollitz.pdf.

Kohrman, Arthur F. 1991. "Medical Technology: Implications for Health and Social Service Providers." In *The Medically Complex Child: The Transition to Home Care*, edited by Neil J. Hochstadt and Diane M. Yost, 3–13. Chur, Switzerland: Harwood Academic.

Korczynski, Marek. 2003. "Communities of Coping: Collective Emotional Labour in Service Work." *Organization* 10 (1): 55–79.

Lawler, Jocalyn. 1991. *Behind the Screens: Nursing, Somology, and the Problem of the Body*. Melbourne: Churchill Livingstone.

Lawton, Julia. 2003. "Lay Experiences of Health and Illness: Past Research and Future Agendas." *Sociology of Health & Illness* 25 (3): 23–40.

Lehoux, Pascale, Jocelyne Saint-Arnaud, and Lucie Richard. 2004. "The Use of Technology at Home: What Patient Manuals Say and Sell vs. What Patients Face and Fear." *Sociology of Health & Illness* 26 (5): 617–44.

Leidner, Robin. 1993. *Fast Food, Fast Talk: Service Work and the Routinization of Everyday Life*. Berkeley: University of California Press.

Leidner, Robin. 1999. "Emotional Labor in Service Work." *Annals of the American Academy of Political and Social Science* 561:81–95.

Leonard, B., J. D. Brust, and J. J. Sapienza. 1992. "Financial and Time Costs to Parents of Severely Disabled Children." *Public Health Reports* 107 (3): 302–12.

Leppänen, Vesa. 2008. "Coping with Troublesome Clients in Home Care." *Qualitative Health Research* 18 (9): 1195–205.

Levine, Carol. 2006. "A Caregiver's Assessment of Assessments: Accused, Tried, and Convicted of Unspecified Crimes against Authority." *American Journal of Nursing* 106 (8): 43.

Levine, Carol. 2008. "Supporting Family Caregivers: Needed; Nursing and Social Work Leadership." *American Journal of Nursing* 108 (9): 13–15.

Levitsky, Sandra R. 2008. " 'What Rights?' The Construction of Political Claims to American Health Care Entitlements." *Law & Society Review* 42 (3): 551–89.

Lewis, Patricia. 2005. "Suppression or Expression: An Exploration of Emotion Management in a Special Care Baby Unit." *Work, Employment and Society* 19 (3): 565–81.

Lindhardt, Tove, Ingrid A. Bolmsjö, and Ingalill Rahm Hallberg. 2006. "Standing Guard—Being a Relative to a Hospitalized, Elderly Person." *Journal of Aging Studies* 20:133–49.

Lively, Kathryn J. 2013. "Social and Cultural Influencers: Gender Effects on Emotional Labor at Work and at Home." In *Emotional Labor in the 21st Century: Diverse Perspectives on Emotion Regulation at Work*, edited by Alicia A. Grandey, James M. Diefendorff, and Deborah E. Rupp, 223–49. New York: Routledge.

Lively, Kathryn J., Lala Carr Steelman, and Brian Powell. 2010. "Equity, Emotion, and Household Division of Labor Response." *Social Psychology Quarterly* 73 (4): 358–79.

Lopez, Steven H. 2004. *Reorganizing the Rust Belt: An Inside Study of the American Labor Movement*. Berkeley: University of California Press.

Lopez, Steven H. 2006. "Emotional Labor and Organized Emotional Care: Conceptualizing Nursing Home Work." *Work and Occupations* 33 (2): 133–60.

Lopez, Steven H. 2010. "Workers, Managers, and Customers: Triangles of Power in Work Communities." *Work and Occupations* 37 (3): 251–71.

Lorber, Judith. 1994. *Paradoxes of Gender*. New Haven, CT: Yale University Press.

Luker, Karen A., Lynn Austin, Ann Caress, and Christine E. Hallett. 2000. "The Importance of 'Knowing the Patient': Community Nurses' Constructions of Quality in Providing Palliative Care." *Journal of Advanced Nursing* 31 (4): 775–82.

Mac Rae, Hazel 1998. "Managing Feelings: Caregiving as Emotion Work." *Research on Aging* 20 (1): 137–60.

Macdonald, Cameron L. 2008. "High-Tech Home Care: Family Caregivers and Consequences." Paper presented at the plenary session at the Annual Meeting of the American Sociological Association, Boston, August 1–4, 2008.

Macdonald, Cameron L. 2010. *Shadow Mothers: Nannies, Au Pairs, and the Micropolitics of Mothering*. Berkeley: University of California Press.

Malat, Jennifer, and Mary Ann Hamilton. 2006. "Preference for Same-Race Health Care Providers and Perceptions of Interpersonal Discrimination in Health Care." *Journal of Health and Social Behavior* 47 (2): 173–87.

Marrone, Catherine. 2003. "Home Health Care Nurses' Perceptions of Physician-Nurse Relationships." *Qualitative Health Research* 13 (5): 623–35.

Mayall, Berry. 1993. "Keeping Children Healthy: The Intermediate Domain." *Social Science & Medicine* 36 (1): 77–83.

Mayes, Rick, and Robert A. Berenson. 2006. *Medicare Prospective Payment and the Shaping of U.S. Health Care*. Baltimore: Johns Hopkins University Press.

McGuire, Gail M. 2007. "Intimate Work: A Typology of the Social Support That Workers Provide to Their Network Members." *Work and Occupations* 34 (2): 125–47.

McKeever, Patricia. 1999. "Between Women: Nurses and Family Caregivers." *Canadian Journal of Nursing Research* 30 (4): 185–91.

Medicare. 2011. "Glossary." http://www.medicare.gov/Glossary/search.asp?SelectAlphabet=S&Language=English (site discontinued).

Messias, Deanne K. Hilfinger, Eun-Ok Im, Aroha Page, Hanna Regev, Judith Spiers, Laurie Yoder, and Afaf Ibrahim Meleis. 1997. "Defining and Redefining Work: Implications for Women's Health." *Gender & Society* 11 (3): 296–323.

Meyer, Madonna Harrington, Pam Herd, and Sonya Michel. 2000. "Introduction: The Right to—or Not to—Care." In *Care Work: Gender, Labor and the Welfare State*, edited by Madonna Harrington Meyer, 1–4. New York: Routledge.

Michelson, William, and Lorne Tepperman. 2003. "Focus on Home: What Time-Use Data Can Tell about Caregiving to Adults." *Journal of Social Issues* 59 (3): 591–610.

Mills, C. Wright. 1959. *The Sociological Imagination*. Oxford: Oxford University Press.

Moeller, Philip. 2013. "Why Caregivers Are an Endangered Species." *USA Today*, September 4, 2013.

Moorman, Sara M., and Cameron Macdonald. 2012. "Medically Complex Home Care and Caregiver Strain." *Gerontologist* 53 (3): 407–17.

Morris, Marika. 2004. "What Research Reveals about Gender, Home Care, and Caregiving: Overview and the Case for Gender Analysis." In *Caring For/Caring About: Women, Home Care and Unpaid Caregiving*, edited by Karen R. Grant, Carol Amaratunga, Pat Armstrong, Madeline Boscoe, Ann Pederson, and Kay Willson, 91–113. Aurora, ON: Garamond.

Murphy, Kathleen E. 1991. "Stress and Coping in Home Care: A Study of Families." In *The Medically Complex Child: The Transition to Home Care*, edited by Neil J. Hochstadt and Diane M. Yost, 287–302. Chur, Switzerland: Harwood Academic.

NAC (National Alliance for Caregiving) and AARP. 2009. *Caregiving in the U.S. 2009*. Bethesda, MD: NAC. November 2009. https://www.caregiving.org/data/Caregiving_in_the_US_2009_full_report.pdf.

NAC (National Alliance for Caregiving) and AARP. 2015. *Executive Summary: Caregiving in the U.S. 2015*. Bethesda, MD: NAC. June 2015. https://www.caregiving.org/wp-content/uploads/2015/05/2015_CaregivingintheUS_Executive-Summary-June-4_WEB.pdf.

NAC (National Alliance for Caregiving) and Evercare. 2007. *Evercare Study of Family Caregivers—What They Spend, What They Sacrifice: The Personal Financial Toll of Caring for a Loved One*. Bethesda, MD: NAC. November 2007. http://www.caregiving.org/data/Evercare_NAC_CaregiverCostStudyFINAL20111907.pdf.

NAHC (National Association for Home Care and Hospice). 2008. *Basic Statistics about Home Care*. Washington, DC: NAHC. http://www.nahc.org/facts/08HC_Stats.pdf (site discontinued).

NAHC (National Association for Home Care and Hospice). 2019. "NAHC Advocacy." https://www.nahc.org/advocacy-policy/.

NCSBN (National Council of State Boards of Nursing). 2011a. "Duties of Boards of Nursing." https://www.ncsbn.org/boards.htm (site discontinued).

NCSBN (National Council of State Boards of Nursing). 2011b. *NCSBN Model Nursing Practice Act and Model Nursing Administrative Rules*. Chicago: NCSB. https://www. ncsbn.org/Model_Practice_Act_March2011.pdf (site discontinued).

NCSL (National Conference of State Legislatures). 2018. "State Insurance Mandates and the ACA Essential Benefits Provisions." http://www.ncsl.org/research/health/ state-ins-mandates-and-aca-essential-benefits.aspx.

NHPF (National Health Policy Forum). 2013. *The Basics: The Commission on Long-Term Care; Background behind the Mission*. Washington, DC: George Washington University. October 17, 2013. http://www.nhpf.org/library/the-basics/Basics_Com missionLTC_10-17-13.pdf.

Noddings, Nel. 1995. "Moral Obligation or Moral Support for High-Tech Home Care?" In *Bringing the Hospital Home*, edited by John D. Arras, 149–65. Baltimore: Johns Hopkins University Press.

NPWF (National Partnership for Women and Families). 2019. *The Family and Medical Insurance Leave (FAMILY) Act Fact Sheet*. Washington, DC: NPWF. February 2019. http://www.nationalpartnership.org/our-work/resources/workplace/paid-leave/family-act-fact-sheet.pdf.

NRSCIS (Northwest Regional Spinal Cord Injury System). 2011. "Taking Care of Your Bowels: The Basics." Seattle: SCI Clinics, Harborview Medical Center and University of Washington Medical Center. http://sci.washington.edu/info/pamphlets/bow els_1.asp.

Ogburn, William F. 1922. *Social Change with Respect to Culture and Original Nature*. New York: Huebsch.

Okun, Alex. 1995. "The History of Respirators and Total Parenteral Nutrition in the Home and Their Use in Children Today." In *Bringing the Hospital Home*, edited by John D. Arras, 35–52. Baltimore: Johns Hopkins University Press.

Oliver, Judith. 1983. "The Caring Wife." In *A Labour of Love: Women, Work and Caring*, edited by Janet Finch and Dulcie Groves, 72–88. London: Routledge and Kegan Paul.

Osmond, Marie Withers, and Barrie Thorne. 1993. "Feminist Theories: The Social Construction of Gender in Families and Society." In *Sourcebook of Family Theories and Methods: A Contextual Approach*, edited by Pauline G. Boss, William J. Doherty, Ralph LaRossa, Walter R. Schumm, and Suzanne K. Steinmetz, 591–625. New York: Plenum.

Oudshoorn, Abram, Catherine Ward-Griffin, and Carol McWilliam. 2007. "Client-Nurse Relationships in Home-Based Palliative Care: A Critical Analysis of Power Relations." *Journal of Clinical Nursing* 16 (8): 1435–43.

Padavic, Irene, and Barbara Reskin. 2002. *Women and Men at Work: Sociology for a New Century*. 2nd ed. Thousand Oaks, CA: Sage.

Pear, Robert. 2018. " 'Short Term' Health Insurance? Up to 3 Years under New Trump Policy." *New York Times*, August 1, 2018.

Pew Research Center. 2011. "Public Wants Changes in Entitlements, Not Changes in Benefits: GOP Divided over Benefit Reductions." July 7, 2011. http://www.people-press.org/2011/07/07/public-wants-changes-in-entitlements-not-change-in-benefits/.

Phillips, Melanie. 2011. "The Real Reason Our Hospitals Are a Disgrace." *Daily Mail*, October 17, 2011. http://www.dailymail.co.uk/debate/article-2049906/How-femi nism-nurses-grand-care.htm.

Piercy, Kathleen W., and Gregory J. Dunkley. 2004. "What Quality Paid Home Care Means to Family Caregivers." *Journal of Applied Gerontology* 23 (3): 175–92.

Piercy, Kathleen W., and Dorothy N. Woolley. 1999. "Negotiating Worker-Client Relationships: A Necessary Step to Providing Quality Home Health Care." *Home Health Care Services Quarterly* 18 (1): 1–24.

Pinquart, M., and S. Sörensen. 2007. "Correlates of Physical Health of Informal Caregivers: A Meta-Analysis." *Journals of Gerontology, Series B, Psychological Sciences and Social Sciences* 62 (2): 126–37.

Porter, Sam. 1992a. "The Poverty of Professionalization: A Critical Analysis of Strategies for the Occupational Advancement of Nursing." *Journal of Advanced Nursing* 17 (6): 720–26.

Porter, Sam. 1992b. "Women in a Women's Job: The Gendered Experience of Nurses." *Sociology of Health & Illness* 14 (4): 510–27.

Porterfield, Shirley. 2004. "Work Choices of Mothers in Families with Children with Disabilities." *Journal of Marriage and Family* 64:972–81.

Prior, Lindsay. 2003. "Belief, Knowledge and Expertise: The Emergence of the Lay Expert in Medical Sociology." *Sociology of Health & Illness* 25 (3): 41–57.

Reed, Jessica. 2012. "Is Nursing Lacking in Compassion?" *Guardian* (US edition), December 4, 2012. http://www.theguardian.com/commentisfree/2012/dec/04/is-nursing-lacking-in-compassion.

Reinhard, Susan C., Carol Levine, and Sarah Samis. 2012. *Home Alone: Family Caregivers Providing Complex Chronic Care.* Washington, DC: AARP Public Policy Institute. October 2012. https://www.aarp.org/content/dam/aarp/research/public_policy_institute/health/home-alone-family-caregivers-providing-complex-chronic-care-rev-AARP-ppi-health.pdf.

Reinhard, Susan C., Heather M. Young, Carol Levine, Kathleen Kelly, Rita B. Choula, and Jean C. Accius. 2019. *Home Alone Revisited: Family Caregivers Providing Complex Care.* Washington, DC: AARP Public Policy Institute. April 2019. https://www.aarp.org/content/dam/aarp/ppi/2019/04/home-alone-revisited-family-caregivers-providing-complex-care.pdf.

Reinhard, Susan C., Heather M. Young, Elaine Ryan, and Rita B. Choula. 2019. *The CARE Act Implementation: Progress and Promise.* Washington, DC: AARP Public Policy Institute. March 2019. https://www.aarp.org/content/dam/aarp/ppi/2019/03/the-care-act-implementation-progress-and-promise.pdf.

Rice, Robyn. 2006a. *Home Care Nursing Practice: Concepts and Application.* Saint Louis, MO: Mosby Elsevier.

Rice, Robyn. 2006b. "The Ventilator Dependent Patient." In Rice, *Home Care Nursing Practice*, 216–39.

Rice, Robyn, Laurel Wiersema-Bryant, and Jackie Bangert. 2006. "The Patient with Chronic Wounds." In Rice, *Home Care Nursing Practice*, 240–67.

Risman, Barbara J. 2004. "Gender as a Social Structure: Theory Wrestling with Activism." *Gender & Society* 18 (4): 429–50.

Rose, Miriam S., Linda S. Noelker, and Jill Kagan. 2015. "Improving Policies for Caregiver Respite Services." *Gerontologist* 55 (2): 302–8.

Roy, Donald F. 1952. "Quota Restriction and Goldbricking in a Machine Shop." *American Journal of Sociology* 57 (5): 427–42.

Salvage, Jane. 1992. "The New Nursing: Empowering Patients or Empowering Nurses?" In *Policy Issues in Nursing*, edited by Jane Robinson, Alastair Gray, and Ruth Elkan, 9–23. Milton Keynes: Open University Press.

Schulz, Richard, and Scott R. Beach. 1999. "Caregiving as a Risk Factor for Mortality: The Caregiver Health Effects Study." *JAMA* 282 (23): 2215–19.

Schulz, Richard, Alison T. O'Brien, Jamila Bookwala, and Kathy Fleissner. 1995. "Psychiatric and Physical Morbidity Effects of Caregiving: Prevalence, Correlates, and Causes." *Gerontologist* 35 (6): 771–91.

Scott, Ellen K. 2010. "I Feel As If I Am the One Who Is Disabled." *Gender & Society* 24 (5): 672–96.

Sherman, Rachel. 2007. *Class Acts: Service and Inequality in Luxury Hotels*. Berkeley: University of California Press.

Simmons, Bret L., Debra L. Nelson, and Leslie Jean Neal. 2001. "A Comparison of the Positive and Negative Work Attitudes of Home Health Care and Hospital Nurses." *Health Care Management Review* 26 (3): 63–74.

Smith, Dorothy. 1987. *The Everyday World as Problematic: A Feminist Sociology*. Boston: Northeastern University Press.

Smith, Leon G., and Michael M. Rothkopf. 1992. "Intravenous Antibiotics." In *Intensive Home Care*, edited by Michael M. Rothkopf and Jeffrey Askanazi, 95–108. Baltimore: Williams and Wilkins.

Smith, Pam. 1991. "The Nursing Process: Raising the Profile of Emotional Care in Nursing Training." *Journal of Advanced Nursing* 16:74–81.

Sörensen, Silvia, Martin Pinquart, and Paul Duberstein. 2002. "How Effective Are Interventions with Caregivers? An Updated Meta-analysis." *Gerontologist* 42 (3): 356–72.

Stacey, Clare L. 2005. "Finding Dignity in Dirty Work: The Constraints and Rewards of Low-Wage Home Care Labour." *Sociology of Health & Illness* 27 (6): 831–54.

Stacey, Clare L. 2011. *The Caring Self: The Work Experiences of Home Care Aides*. Ithaca, NY: Cornell University Press.

Stacey, Clare L., and Lindsey L. Ayers. 2012. "Caught between Love and Money: The Experiences of Paid Family Caregivers." *Qualitative Sociology* 35:47–64.

Stacey, M., and C. Davies. 1983. *Division of Labour in Child Health Care*. London: Economic and Social Research Council.

Stone, Deborah. 2001. "Care and Trembling." *American Prospect*, November 16. https://prospect.org/health/care-trembling/.

Strauss, Anselm, Shizuko Fagerhaugh, Barbara Suczek, and Carolyn Wiener. 1982. "Sentimental Work in the Technological Hospital." *Sociology of Health & Illness* 4 (3): 255–78.

ten Hoeve, Yvonne, Gerard Jansen, and Petrie Roodbol. 2013. "The Nursing Profession: Public Image, Self-Concept and Professional Identity; A Discussion Paper." *Journal of Advanced Nursing* 70 (2), 295–309.

Theodosius, Catherine. 2008. *Emotional Labour in Health Care: The Unmanaged Heart of Nursing.* London: Routledge.

Thoits, P. A. 1996. "Managing the Emotions of Others." *Symbolic Interaction* 19:85–109.

Thorne, Barrie. 1992. "Feminism and the Family: Two Decades of Thought." In *Rethinking the Family: Some Feminist Questions,* edited by Barrie Thorne and Marilyn Yalom, 3–30. Boston: Northeastern University Press.

Tolich, Martin B. 1993. "Alienating and Liberating Emotions at Work: Supermarket Clerks' Performance of Customer Service." *Journal of Contemporary Ethnography* 22 (3): 361–81.

Tronto, Joan. 1993. *Moral Boundaries: A Political Argument for an Ethic of Care.* New York: Routledge, Chapman and Hall.

Twigg, Julia. 1999. "The Spatial Ordering of Care: Public and Private in Bathing Support at Home." *Sociology of Health & Illness* 21 (4): 381–400.

Twigg, Julia. 2000. "Carework as a Form of Bodywork." *Ageing and Society* 20:389–411.

Twigg, Julia, Carol Wolkowitz, Rachel Lara Cohen, and Sarah Nettleton. 2011. "Conceptualising Body Work in Health and Social Care." *Sociology of Health & Illness* 33 (2): 171–88.

Ungerson, Clare. 1983. "Why Do Women Care?" In *A Labour of Love: Women, Work and Caring,* edited by Janet Finch and Dulcie Groves, 31–49. London: Routledge and Kegan Paul.

Ungerson, Clare. 1987. *Policy Is Personal: Sex, Gender, and Informal Care.* London: Tavistock.

Ungerson, Clare. 1990a. Introduction to *Gender and Caring: Work and Welfare in Britain and Scandinavia,* edited by Clare Ungerson, 1–7. New York: Harvester Wheatsheaf.

Ungerson, Clare. 1990b. "The Language of Care: Crossing the Boundaries." In *Gender and Caring: Work and Welfare in Britain and Scandinavia,* edited by Clare Ungerson, 8–33. New York: Harvester Wheatsheaf.

U.S. Census Bureau. 2010. "Health Insurance Coverage Status and Type of Coverage—All Persons by Sex, Race and Hispanic Origin: 1999 to 2009." http://www.census.gov/hhes/www/hlthins/data/historical/files/hihistt1.xls (site discontinued).

U.S. Census Bureau. 2013. *Income, Poverty, and Health Insurance Coverage in the United States.* Washington, DC: U.S. Census Bureau. September 2013. http://www.census.gov/prod/2013pubs/p60-245.pdf.

USDHHS (U.S. Department of Health and Human Services). 2013. Administration on Aging. "Aging Statistics—Profile of Older Americans." http://www.aoa.gov/AoARoot/Aging_Statistics/Profile/index.aspx (site discontinued).

USDHHS (U.S. Department of Health and Human Services). 2018. "About the Affordable Care Act." https://www.hhs.gov/healthcare/about-the-aca/index.html.

USDOL (U.S. Department of Labor). 2014. Bureau of Labor Statistics. "Healthcare: Millions of Jobs Now and in the Future." *Occupational Outlook Quarterly,* Spring 2014. https://www.bls.gov/careeroutlook/2014/spring/art03.pdf.

USDOL (U.S. Department of Labor). 2019. "FMLA (Family and Medical Leave)." https://www.dol.gov/general/topic/benefits-leave/fmla.

USNLM (U.S. National Library of Medicine, National Institutes of Health). 2011a. "MedlinePlus: Changing Your Ostomy Pouch." http://www.nlm.nih.gov/medline plus/ency/patientinstrutions/000204.htm (site discontinued).

USNLM (U.S. National Library of Medicine, National Institutes of Health). 2011b. "MedlinePlus: Percutaneous Urinary Procedures." http://www.nlm.nih.gov/medline plus/ency/article/007375.htm.

USNLM (U.S. National Library of Medicine. National Institutes of Health). 2011c. "MedlinePlus: Spasticity." http://www.nlm.nih.gov/medlineplus/ency/article/003297.htm.

USNLM (U.S. National Library of Medicine, National Institutes of Health). 2011d. "MedlinePlus: Urinary Catheters." http://www.nlm.nih.gov/medlineplus/ency/article/ 003981.htm.

USNLM (U.S. National Library of Medicine, National Institutes of Health). 2011e. "MedlinePlus: Wet to Dry Dressing Changes." http://www.nlm.nih.gov/medlineplus/ ency/patientinstrutions/000315.htm (site discontinued).

USNLM (U.S. National Library of Medicine, National Institutes of Health). 2018. "MedlinePlus: Ostomy." http://www.nlm.nih.gov/medlineplus/ostomy.html.

USNLM (U.S. National Library of Medicine. National Institutes of Health). 2019. MedlinePlus: *Daily Bowel Care Program*. Bethesda, MD: USNLM. https://medline plus.gov/ency/patientinstructions/000133.htm.

USVA (U.S. Department of Veterans Affairs). 2019a. Geriatrics and Extended Care. "Veteran Directed Care." https://www.va.gov/geriatrics/guide/longtermcare/veteran-directed_care.asp#.

USVA (U.S. Department of Veterans Affairs). 2019b. Pension. "Aid & Attendance and Housebound." https://www.benefits.va.gov/pension/aid_attendance_housebound.asp.

USVA (U.S. Department of Veterans Affairs). 2019c. "The Program of Comprehensive Assistance for Family Caregivers." https://www.va.gov/health-care/family-care giver-benefits/comprehensive-assistance/.

USVA (U.S. Department of Veterans Affairs). 2019d. VA Caregiver Support. "Mission Act." https://www.caregiver.va.gov/.

UW Health (University of Wisconsin Hospital). 2010. "Health Information: Health Facts for You." http://uwhealth.org/healthfacts/b_extranet_health_information-fex member-show_public_hffy_1108423940681.html (site discontinued).

Wærness, Kari. 1978. "The Invisible Welfare State: Women's Work at Home." Special Congress issue, *Acta Sociologica*, 21:193–207.

Wakabayashi, Chizuko, and Katharine M. Donato. 2006. "Does Caregiving Increase Poverty among Women in Later Life? Evidence from the Health and Retirement Study." *Journal of Health and Social Behavior* 47:258–74.

Walker, Alexis J., Clara C. Pratt, and Linda Eddy. 1995. "Informal Caregiving to Aging Family Members: A Critical Review." *Family Relations* 44 (4): 402–11.

Ward-Griffin, Catherine, and Victor W. Marshall. 2003. "Reconceptualizing the Relationship between 'Public' and 'Private' Eldercare." *Journal of Aging Studies* 17: 189–208.

Wharton, Amy S. 1993. "The Affective Consequences of Service Work: Managing Emotions on the Job." *Work and Occupations* 20 (2): 203–32.

Wiles, Janine. 2003. "Daily Geographies of Caregivers: Mobility, Routine, Scale." *Social Science & Medicine* 57 (7): 1307–25.

Williams, Allison. 2002. "Changing Geographies of Care: Employing the Concept of Therapeutic Landscapes as a Framework in Examining Home Space." *Social Science & Medicine* 55 (1): 141–54.

Williams, Brian, Joanne Coyle, and David Healy. 1998. "The Meaning of Patient Satisfaction: An Explanation of High Reported Levels." *Social Science & Medicine* 47 (9): 1351–59.

Williams, Claire. 2000. "Alert Assistants in Managing Chronic Illness: The Case of Mothers and Teenage Sons." *Sociology of Health & Illness* 22 (2): 254–72.

Williams, Gareth. 1984. "The Genesis of Chronic Illness: Narrative Reconstruction." *Sociology of Health & Illness* 6 (2): 175–200.

Wolkowitz, Carol. 2006. *Bodies at Work*. London: Sage.

Wright, Eric R., and Brea L. Perry. 2010. "Medical Sociology and Health Services Research: Past Accomplishments and Future Policy Changes." *Journal of Health and Social Behavior* 51:S107–18.

Wright, Mareena McKinley. 1995. "'I Never Did Any Fieldwork, but I Milked an Awful Lot of Cows!' Using Rural Women's Experience to Reconceptualize Models of Work." *Gender & Society* 9 (2): 216–35.

Wrobleski, Diane Salentiny, M. Ellen Joswiak, Donna F. Dunn, Pamela M. Maxson, and Diane E. Holland. 2014. "Discharge Planning Rounds to the Bedside: A Patient- and Family-Centered Approach." *Medsurg Nursing* 23 (2): 111–16.

Yantzi, Nicole M., and Mark W. Rosenberg. 2008. "The Contested Meanings of Home for Women Caring for Children with Long-Term Needs in Ontario, Canada." *Gender, Place and Culture* 15 (3): 301–15.

Zarit, Steven H., Karen E. Reever, and Julie Bach-Peterson. 1980. "Relatives of the Impaired Elderly: Correlates of Feelings of Burden." *Gerontologist* 20 (6): 649–55.

Zelizer, Viviana A. 2005. *The Purchase of Intimacy*. Princeton, NJ: Princeton University Press.

INDEX

CPSIA information can be obtained
at www.ICGtesting.com
Printed in the USA
LVHW100448051122
732387LV00004B/401

9 781501 751455